Intellectual Disability

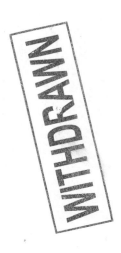

Intellectual Disability

Social Approaches

David Race

Open University Press

Open University Press
McGraw-Hill Education
McGraw-Hill House
Shoppenhangers Road
Maidenhead
Berkshire
England
SL6 2QL

email: enquiries@openup.co.uk
world wide web: www.openup.co.uk

and Two Penn Plaza, New York, NY 10121-2289, USA

First published 2007

A catalogue record of this book is available from the British Library

ISBN-978 0335 22136 3 (pb) 978 0335 22137 0 (hb)
ISBN-0 335 22136 X (pb) 0 335 22137 8 (hb)

Library of Congress Cataloging-in-Publication Data
CIP data applied for

Typeset by RefineCatch Limited, Bungay, Suffolk
Printed in Poland EU, by OZgraf S.A., www.polskabook.pl

The *McGraw·Hill* Companies

In memory of Jennifer Lewis, 1950–2004.

For bringing me to Debbie, us to the world
of intellectual disability, and light to the lives of
all who met her.

Contents

List of figures and tables

Figures

Tables

Foreword

John O'Brien

The Center on Human Policy, Syracuse University

David Race and I have each had the privilege of belonging to an international network committed to reforming services to people with learning difficulties by applying the principle of normalization, as defined by Wolf Wolfensberger and later redefined by him as Social Role Valorization (SRV). The principle of normalization was much debated, and even more frequently invoked, through the 1970s and 1980s as shifting patterns of public expenditure, the rising influence of advocates, revulsion at institutional conditions, and a growing base of practical knowledge shaped the growth of community services. This book, based on an around-the-world tour of countries where normalization/ SRV has been influential, offers a comparative account of the ways these ideas have worked out in seven different national contexts more than 30 years after their introduction.

This could have been a triumphant book; instead it is a sober one, and far more useful for it. For every country he visited, David could have written about the sophistication and passion with which people committed to implementing SRV have elaborated the ideas, refined their competence to analyze policy and practice, and strengthened their ability to teach. For every country he visited, David could have written inspiring and informative accounts of the innovations generated by people who have taken SRV seriously and the exceptional and ordinary lives that some people with learning difficulties have because of those innovations. He could have collected postcards of exceptions. Instead, he has carefully built up impressionistic portraits of each nation that suggest the probable experience of ordinary people and families who rely on typically available services.

Each impression portrays similar aspects. David indicates history, background beliefs about welfare and consequent administrative arrangements. He sketches service provision from early childhood through a move out of the family home and indicates the odds that a typical service user at each stage of life will have the opportunity and necessary assistance to take up a valued social role. He highlights how much difference family privilege and family energy make in determining service experiences. He shades in the effects of class, race, and income on the experience of service. All of this is sobering enough – outside the Nordic Countries, the prospects of straightforward access to publicly funded assistance to take up socially valued roles remain discouraging, and even access to service demands significant family effort. Everywhere, opportunities for real jobs are scarce and the chances of being included in ordinary schools go down as need for assistance goes up. The exceptional brightly colored patches – places where services make a strong positive difference to people's life chances – demonstrate that SRV can be powerfully implemented and make the overall grayness of most of the national portraits more frustrating.

But it is the undercoating of most of the portraits that is darkest. Sensitive to the historic power of eugenic ideas that cast people with learning difficulties as, more than worthless, positively dangerous to society, ideas that captured many progressive thinkers early in the last century, David outlines the influence of eugenics on the development of each nation's services. Then, most sobering of all this book's messages, he shows the continuing power of eugenic ideas by considering the chances that a person with a disability detectable before birth will be born at all. In more nations than not, the odds against being born disabled rise steadily.

Thoughtfully preparing each national portrait and considering the differences among them disclosed an important insight. In the English-speaking countries portrayed in this book, the way people make sense of services has shifted fundamentally. David calls this shift in social imagination 'managerialism'. Power to allocate resources has passed from people seen to be knowledgeable about people with learning difficulties to people seen to be knowledgeable about managing budgets against abstractions like 'value for money'. Judgements of value are based on scattered assumptions about which professionally delivered practices are supported as cost-effective by abstract evidence rather than on a coherent understanding about how services can assist people to occupy a valued social role and thus experience the ordinary good things in life. Quality means producing appropriate documentation of progress toward vague and shifting conceptual targets ('modernizing day services' or 'improving delivery on outcomes') rather than learning to improve the concrete dimensions of daily life indicated by SRV. The notions attached to the market state – in which the identity of persons fulfilled by many social roles collapses into the role of service consumer for whom choice (within limits that minimize state expenditure) is the supreme good – provide the vocabulary for understanding, influencing, and implementing policy.

Within this disorienting horizon, important ideas like SRV can help committed people find their bearings. But these ideas lose their power because they no longer fit within common terms of sense-making and thus they cannot guide practical action. Their function thins to slogans cut and pasted if a document needs decoration. It is only in enclaves that purposely keep alive the language and the practices necessary to make sense of them that people will be able to draw on the demonstrated power of SRV ideas. As this book makes clear, these enclaves are harder to create today than they were 30 years ago, and even more necessary.

This book is sober and thoughtful; David's impressions set our feet on the ground. And, as the reader will find as the final chapter chronicles the lessons of the traveler's homecoming, it is ultimately quietly hopeful and quietly joyful.

Acknowledgements

Far more people have made significant contributions to this book than I can possibly acknowledge, which is a source of some regret. They will be aware, however, of their impact on the world described herein, and I hope at least they feel I have represented something of its subtleties.

To my hosts in the various countries, not just for their company and hospitality, but also the stimulation of their views, and their efforts to put me in touch with significant people, I give many thanks. Still more to those of them who offered comments and corrections to the draft chapters on their respective countries. In the order of the chapters, they are Eva-Lena Kall, from Sweden; Karl-Johan Johansen and Kristjana Kristiansen from Norway; Lorna Sullivan and Steph Roberts from New Zealand; Margaret Spalding, Greg Mackay, Jane Sherwin, Errol Cocks and Eddie Tse from Australia; Zana Lutfiyya, Bill Foreman and Judith Sandys from Canada; and Steve Taylor, Marc Tumeinski, Jo Massarelli, Debi Reidy, Michael Kendrick and Jack Yates from the USA.

To John O'Brien, not only for his Foreword, but for continuing encouragement throughout the writing of the book, not least his tolerance of my early attempts to hack my way through the jungle of the US service system, I am deeply grateful. Needless to say, especially to John, all those people are not responsible for the final version, which is in my hands, but none of it would have been possible without them. Nor would it without the support from my School at Salford University, Community, Health Sciences and Social Care, especially the Head, Karen Kniveton, for their policy of study leave, and to Rachel Gear, at McGraw-Hill and Open University Press, for agreeing to publish the results of that study leave, and for tolerance of the other demands on my time in terms of flexible deadlines. The support of my colleagues on the learning disability team at Salford, in covering for me over the five months, should also be acknowledged, as should the university's Research Investment Fund, for their contribution to my costs.

My colleague Angela Olsen, who did a great deal of the statistical research for Chapter 1, is also due my gratitude, with the hope that this will encourage her to develop further her considerable potential as a researcher.

As for my wife Debbie, who not only developed Angela's work, but put my totally haphazard system of referencing into order, the mere expression of thanks seems inadequate, since those tasks, brilliantly as she did them, are but a tiny part of the debt I owe to her, some of which may become apparent to readers as they go through the book.

Finally, to my son Adam, who is actually the real star of the book, thanks are due not only for his customary willingness, indeed enthusiasm, for me to talk and write about his life, but also simply for that life. All my four sons have brought the usual parental mixture of pride, joy, anger and sorrow, and Adam's brothers, in making him part of our family, continue to have our thanks, but the man himself, by developing into, in the words of a local expression, a 'grand lad', affirms both my life and work, including this modest offering.

David Race
Salford and Chelmorton
January 2007

Introduction
A personal approach

'You are old, Father William', the young man said, 'and your hair is exceedingly white, and yet you increasingly stand on your head, do you think, at your age, this is right?'

(Lewis Carroll)

This has been the most enjoyable, and yet the most difficult, book I have attempted in thirty years of academic writing. Most enjoyable, if I include in the process my five months study leave visiting the six countries that, with my own, make up the 'social approaches' to intellectual disability services described and discussed in succeeding chapters. More so if I include earlier visits to some of those countries stretching back over 30 years.

Most difficult for much the same reason, however, is the humbling and daunting task of attempting to do justice to the many hours of discussion and debate with people, as well as the unique access they afforded me to examples of services and both published and more informal literature. 'Standing on my head' is therefore a minor accomplishment by comparison, and yet such a notion could describe the experience of writing what follows, in that what I hope has emerged is a look from a variety of angles at the countries' intellectual disability services. Those angles are peculiar to me in the sense that, to mix metaphors, the head on which I was standing to observe and discuss wore a number of different hats. As an academic, certainly, but also as a parent of someone with an intellectual disability, a member of an international network, perhaps even a movement, to try and influence services to help people have better lives, and someone whose hair, though not 'exceedingly white', is grey enough to signify a longish history in all those endeavours.

So a personal approach to 'social approaches'. This may disappoint those expecting the book to be something that it is not, and it would perhaps be as well to relieve them of their disappointment before they get too much further. This book is *not* an objective, empirically based, comparative study of intellectual disability services. Even if such a thing were possible, which from my particular methodological stance I would doubt, the degree of information and amount of time needed to be spent on even the briefest such study would be prohibitive.

Nor is this book a collection of 'good stories', of exciting new approaches brought back by the traveller to amaze the modern equivalent of the Royal Geographical Society. Reference will be made to interesting experiences and people I met, and there will be examples of, or at least reference to, what might be considered 'good' or 'radical' services, but this is not a search for the holy service grail. It *is* important to compare countries in terms of the radical things they are doing, or are trying to do, and I have come across all too few publications that do so (two that have been extremely useful to me are Johnson and Traustadottir, 2005 and O'Brien and Murray, 1997) but that is not my purpose here.

Nor still is this book an attempt to use the observations of the different countries to construct some sort of a 'theory of services' or 'theory of intellectual disability'. Other attempts at such development of ideas have been very important, especially, from my perspective, both the original formulations of normalization (Nirje 1969; Wolfensberger 1972) and its development into the theory of Social Role Valorization (hereafter SRV) (Wolfensberger 1998; Race 2003), as well as other derivations and developments from those sources, e.g. O'Brien and O'Brien (2000), O'Brien (2005a), Westcott (2003). My own limitations as a theoretician, however, and, more importantly, my desire to orient this book towards families and others involved with services, as well as students and others from the academic field of intellectual disability, have led me away from such an approach.

So what *is* this book trying to do? The answer to that question, which I repeated many times on my travels, is that I am aiming to give 'an impressionistic picture, rather than a photograph' of the different countries and their services. By definition, therefore, it is *my* impressionist picture, my personal approach to social approaches, and thus both my *perceptions* of services, drawn from direct observation, discussion, and reading, as well as how these are presented in the chapters which follow, will be affected by who I am, and what influences the way I perceive and present things. In the process of writing the book, I have done my best, from a distance, to check on the accuracy of what I claim to be factual statements, but the level of detail of those 'facts', combined with the enormity of information that would be poured out were every specific variation in each country to be listed, means that my descriptions are much more often broad, and couched in terms of impressions and probabilities.

The end result may therefore be, rather than standing on my head, I am falling onto it between stools, so that even those who *do* want what I am trying to convey are disappointed, but I will leave them to be the judge of that. What I will do, however, to give readers a stronger idea of where my impressions are coming from, is to use the framework that comes at the beginning of most presentations and texts on SRV (e.g. Wolfensberger 1998; Race 1999) concerning factors that affect how an observer makes a 'social judgement' on different people or social groups. Those unfamiliar with SRV need not feel at a disadvantage here, since this framework can stand in its own right. The point of using the framework is to set the context for the rest of the book, in which I, as the 'observer', will be describing and commenting on services in the different countries. What affects my perceptions should, I believe, be something the reader is entitled to know at the outset, enabling them to temper what they read with that knowledge. Figure 0.1, adapted from Race (1999: 33), sets out the framework

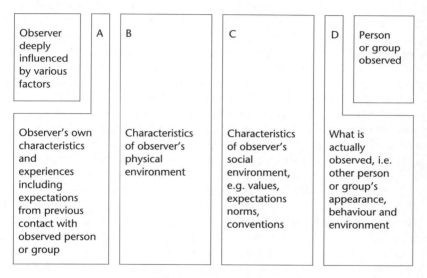

Figure 0.1   Influences on the relativistic social judgement by one person or group on another.

The observer's own characteristics and experiences

This first influence begins with relationships with two people with an intellectual disability, specifically Down's syndrome, linked by a third person who has no impairments, unless her judgement of a partner could be called into question. As I told a number of people on my trip, the reason I became involved at all significantly in this field was the arrival, at the research unit that I had joined after two years in industry following a management degree, of a research assistant with a sister, Jenny, who had Down's syndrome. Immediately one of my range of projects for Berkshire Social Services, to do with 'mental handicap', became much more important, as interest in her sister

Deborah led me to Jenny, to switch my PhD from work on homelessness to intellectual disability and to begin 33 years of involvement with this group of people. For 31 of those years I was to know Jenny as my girl-friend's sister, bridesmaid at my wedding, sister-in-law, aunt to my sons, an example of the power of expectations, and generator of more positive emotions in a whole range of people than I was to see until the arrival in our lives of another person with Down's syndrome. In the 12 years between meeting Jenny and the Christmas of 1985 when Debbie and I adopted Adam, our fourth son, at six months old, my connections and experiences in the field of intellectual disabilities grew significantly. I was then working from home as Consultant (Handicap) for the Children's Society, a national charitable agency, joining in 1983 on my return from Hong Kong University, where I had worked for four years. We had gone out there after two years in a research unit evaluating an 'experiment' in a 'comprehensive service system for the mentally handicapped' in Sheffield. My PhD, completed at Reading University (Race 1977) and a book Debbie and I had written on the first ever group home in England (Race and Race 1979) had taken us to Sheffield, and to a house in the little village in the Peak District of Derbyshire where we still live. Hong Kong expanded the academic side of my work in the field, including the completion of a textbook begun in Sheffield (Malin et al. 1980), but the Children's Society role saw the real expansion of my direct involvement with people with intellectual disabilities and services for them. Work for the Children's Society had also, by the time of Adam's arrival and to some extent contributing to it, enabled me to travel to the USA to attend various events given by Wolf Wolfensberger and his colleagues, as well as making or renewing acquaintance with the network around normalization in the UK. The Children's Society were also responsible for bringing Wolfensberger back to the UK after an absence of 20 years, and events he presented in the 1980s and 1990s began to be organized by a network, which continues to this day, that developed from those early Children's Society workshops.

Adam's story will continue to figure in the book, as will the device of my speculating on his likely life, at its different stages, in the various countries, so that will remain for later, merely noting here its increasing impact on my working life as well as the developing parental experience. One such impact contributed to what I now refer to as my 'masochistic sabbatical', in 1989, when I took a year's training and then served for two years as a primary school teacher on a large deprived public housing estate in the city of Stoke-on-Trent. That period put into perspective what was happening to education and the welfare state in my country at the time, as the full impact of ten years of what has been called 'Thatcherism' began to bite. Then, after a year of being a 'home parent' for most of the time, my next post, teaching on a degree course at what is called a 'College of Further and Higher Education' represented both a decline in income, academic status, and the availability of time to write. Despite this, the international networks continued to flourish, enabling the writing of the first full-length text in English on SRV (Race 1999) and the beginnings of a textbook based on the degree course (Race 2002a), completed after my move to my current post at Salford University in 2000. That move enabled me to increase my academic output, including an edited collection of Wolfensberger's writings (Race 2003) and of course this current book.

So this observer's 'own characteristics and experiences' are as an academic, particularly regarding services for people with intellectual disabilities and normalization/SRV and its derivatives, as someone involved for nearly ten years in the change of a direct service organization (Race and Williams 1988) but above all as someone who has seen and been involved with the real lives of two people with intellectual disabilities.

Running through all this experience, and interacting with it, have been my developing personal beliefs and values, which could be summed up as 'left of centre Christianity'. More recent formal expressions of these beliefs have emerged as I trained from 2003–05 to be a 'Reader' in the Church of England, and the Children's Society experience sought to develop 'faith in action', but the connections between theological and political reflection, and my work and life, go back to my university days, or even earlier. This, too, is part of my 'characteristics and experiences' and has been reinforced by the next element of the 'influences' in Figure 0.1.

Characteristics of observer's physical environment

Though this is usually taken in SRV to refer to the physical environment in which the observation is made, and therefore its effects on the judgement, I will take the liberty of expanding the idea for this book and talk briefly of my 'home' physical environments, as they might relate to my judgement of the physical environments I was visiting. Living for 30 years in a small rural village in England, having lived previously in a similar environment for the two years after my marriage, was a contrast to the physical environments where I lived until I was 18, and for the three years of my undergraduate life. The first was a suburb of London, with daily commuting by train to school, and the second the city of Manchester, though again my actual accommodation was in the suburbs. The point of mentioning this, while less obvious than the social environment which follows, is my view that the physical environment of cities has its own characteristics when it comes to community integration. Class-based geographical areas, with similar accommodation in one place, contrast with the greater variety of accommodation in the small geographical area of a village. Both then are defined by the particularly English style of housing, equally class-defined, generated by population increases and urbanization from the Industrial Revolution of the mid-nineteenth century onwards. My notion of what is an 'ordinary house', therefore, and the amount of space and numbers of people living there will inevitably influence my view on what is presented elsewhere. As we shall see in the next chapter, this is highly related to the population density of my home country, which exceeds all the others in the study.

Characteristics of observer's social environment, e.g. values, expectations norms, conventions

It will be very apparent before readers get to Chapter 8 that massive changes have taken place in English society in my lifetime, partly reflecting global changes but with some peculiar local characteristics of their own. In particular, the deep-rooted class system (e.g. Savage 2000) though much denied or downplayed these days, has impacted massively on me, both positively and negatively. This will be discussed in more detail in Chapter 8 in terms of its effect on services, but in terms of its effect on *me*, two key issues need to be mentioned. My parents would be described as 'lower middle class', my father being a salesman, first in the clothing industry, then of insurance, while my mother, being the intelligent daughter of a family who split up, came to London as a single woman (rare in the 1930s) to work as a tax officer, her parents being unable to afford the cost of her going to university (still rare for a woman at that time). The hopes of the lower middle classes were firmly fixed on their children succeeding in the meritocratic education system brought in after the war, even to the point of paying fees (at considerable sacrifice) for schools that would help with the process. Such parents rarely had the ambition (or sufficient finance) to send their children to the 'public schools' (actually private) that provide the stereotype of the English school system, still reproduced today in Harry Potter's 'Hogwarts', but instead hoped they would obtain a place at one of the newly created 'grammar schools' where roughly 25 per cent of those taking an IQ-based national examination at 11 were placed (Simon 1991). By these means, both my sister and I found ourselves at such schools, expected to perform well enough in the national examinations to get a place at university. To readers from other countries this may sound unremarkable, but the social status of even this relatively elite position bore no comparison with (and elicited far less advantage than) the status of those attending the 'public schools'. As for those selected out by the so-called '11 plus', they were destined for jobs in the burgeoning factories and offices of the 1950s and 1960s, and to struggle to escape the public housing estates where the great majority would live. For people with intellectual disabilities, of course, neither a class nor intellectually based hierarchy put them anywhere special, with the creation of the National Health Service (hereafter NHS) in 1948 (following the 1946 Act of Parliament) firmly placing the institutions into the medical model of care.

That general cultural background fed into the 1960s, and the period of challenge to conventions and institutions that has had such an overblown coverage. It is true that there were changes, not least from a generation of politicians and others who had been through the education system and could see the injustice of what was going on, but for those of us growing to adulthood and into the world of work, the changes did not seem to have been that significant. 'Management' and 'Labour' still thought of themselves in class terms, with Labour and Conservative governments exchanging power in the late 1960s and early 1970s, and the unions generating a series of high profile disputes, to the point where an election was fought on the basis of 'who runs Britain'. Meanwhile, at a social level, class divisions continued in the geographical location of people in the cities and towns, and in the contrast in rural areas between landowners and those working for them.

Moving to a small village in the south of England after getting married in 1974, and then to Derbyshire in 1976 to our current location, Debbie and I, as beneficiaries of the education system, but with a desire to make some use of this for people with intellectual disabilities, were something of an oddity. The Peak District village, when we moved in, had only a couple of people, out of the approximately 360-strong population, who worked any distance from the village, as we were to do in taking the 50-mile round trip to Sheffield. Then, as our first child came along, the much greater social mix of our village became a greater feature of our lives, and this has remained the case ever since, though the Thatcher years produced many other changes in the social environment of England. In particular, the radical approach to unemployment, to the unions, to property, and to the social structure of English society that the Conservative government brought (Clarke 1998) has meant that my current social environment is radically different in many respects to the one that existed when we arrived 30 years ago. In some ways, however, the underlying class assumptions have resurfaced, added to by a new moneyed class, sitting uneasily with the old 'natural leaders' of the public school and 'Oxbridge' elites, but representing the top of a greasy pole of competitive consumerism that will be more familiar to readers from other countries. So my social environment is one which has changed radically, but where the class distinctions I recall from my youth (comically, if incomprehensibly to outsiders, illustrated by the fact that when my school, a 'grammar school', played the famous 'public school' of Eton at cricket, we were not allowed to play their first team, and the second eleven that we did play were not allowed to wear full cricket whites, but played in grey trousers). The obscurity of that example is why it is so hard to explain English (let alone UK) society, but my Englishness needs to be borne in mind when I am commenting on other countries.

What is actually observed

In SRV training, it is usually emphasized that the previous three influences of Figure 0.1 produce a strong predilection to a judgement, even before direct observation is made. I would prefer to say here that they produced a sense, on my part, of what I regard as services likely to make a positive difference in people's lives, and sensitivity to the broader influences from social and physical environments that differ from my own. The first influence, my personal experiences, enabled me to frame questions to people on my visits, and to continually think, and ask, 'What would it be like if Adam were such and such an age here?' My 'observation', then, comes not just, or even mainly, from *direct* personal observation of services, though I did visit quite a number. It also comes from talking to people, and reading a significant amount of literature of all kinds. My background, naturally, influenced to whom I spoke, and therefore readers should be aware that most of my hosts were from the normalization/SRV network. This did not mean I only spoke to people, or observed services, that went along with the ideas of this network, but the significant presence of that group needs to be borne in mind. As do my earlier remarks that this book is not an empirical study of the different countries. Thus there is no claim that services I actually observed were in any way 'representative', rather, that they are examples to lead to discussion. I have also tended to minimize identification of specific places.

The structure of the book

Having outlined the context of the book, it only remains to describe the structure and content. As readers will have already seen from the Contents, this Introduction is followed, in Chapter 1, by a brief historical and demographic overview of the seven countries involved. The next seven chapters provide a detailed impression of each country in turn, with the following structure for each:

- a brief 'Instant Impacts' reflection, of an incident or a person encountered in the country concerned;
- a short history of services in the country;
- an overview, in the form of a summary table, of my impression of the current service system;
- a detailed look at services through the age range, including issues around screening and pre-birth;
- at various points, boxes, headed 'Adam's World Tour', will also be included, with a summary of my views on the likely services Adam

might receive, were he at various points on the age range in the country concerned.

The closing chapter will summarize the 'Adam's World Tour' accounts, followed by conclusions in terms of influences on services that may begin to explain key points of difference between the countries, and ending with a personal reflection.

The order of countries in Chapters 2–8 is, with the exception of England, meant to represent a move from the most comprehensive welfare states, Sweden and Norway, through agency-based services funded and controlled by the national government, in New Zealand, to countries where the different regions of the countries have a greater power and influence over the service system than the national government, but where most services are agency provided. This takes us to Australia, with its specific arrangement between the States and Territories and the national government, to Canada, with almost total Provincial autonomy, and the USA, with its vast differences between different States. England (including reasons why I am talking about England rather than the UK) then forms Chapter 8, placed last partly because it is 'coming home', but also because I include, as well as what might be *expected* to happen by way of services for Adam, what has *actually* happened in his life. This is also the reason why Chapter 8 is slightly longer than the others.

A final point on structure concerns issues that share a common history, or which occur for the first time or more strongly in a particular chapter. These will be discussed as they occur, and then dealt with more briefly in subsequent chapters, with reference back to the initial reflections. In this way it is hoped that the book will have a flow to it, rather than each country's chapter existing in total isolation. We begin with a brief look at the history and demographics of the seven countries.

1   Demographic Overview

'If everybody minded their own business', the Duchess said in a hoarse growl, 'the world would go round a deal faster than it does.'

'Which would not be an advantage', said Alice, who felt very glad to get an opportunity of showing off a little of her knowledge. 'Just think what work it would make with the day and night! You see, the earth takes twenty-four hours to turn round on its axis . . . Twenty-four hours I think; or is it twelve? I . . .'

'Oh, don't bother me', said the Duchess; 'I never could abide figures.'

(Lewis Carroll)

Introduction – the need for a context

Given the rather lengthy justification for the impressionistic style of this book, readers may feel similar sentiments to the Duchess when we start with a chapter containing a high proportion of facts and figures. My response to such a reaction is to continue the notion of an *impression*, and to place before readers, without detailed analysis, some descriptive statistics which may produce speculative insights of an overall nature before the detailed analysis of services in the different countries that follows. I am indebted to my colleague from Salford, Angela Olsen, for her diligent trawling through sources of such information, and the beginnings of its tabulation, and my wife Deborah for continuing the process.

History – countries old and new

The first point of comparison of this chapter raises an issue which reappears several times later, namely the distinction between those countries whose current populations are now dominated numerically by the ancestors of relatively recent settlers/colonizers/immigrants, as compared to those whose indigenous peoples are still a majority. Of course if we go back to pre-history everyone is descended from people who wandered across continental shelves (*National Geographic* 2007). More significant, in terms of who is viewed as 'different', and the power of that view to define difference in terms of devaluation and oppression, is the sense of identity of countries whose majority populations have been on the land for many thousands of years, and those whose majority consists of much more recent arrivals. Especially when those arrivals come from an existing, and long-standing, culture of their own, and are arriving to conquer the new lands, or fleeing from hardship and/or persecution in their homeland, then the mix that evolves over the few hundreds of years is likely to have very different views on 'outsiders' and on who is defined as such.

Space does not permit more than brief speculation on this, but it is a key item in Table 1.1, which gives a (very) brief history of the countries of this book. The order of countries presented in Table 1.1 is the same as the individual chapters, the rationale for which has been given in the Introduction.

Table 1.1 shows the position that will be familiar to most readers, of the three European countries of Sweden, Norway and England still having a majority population that can be called indigenous from pre-history, though with England more mixed. These three European countries can then be contrasted with Australia, Canada and the USA, whose pre-historical populations are far from being in a majority now, or from being in any significant position of power. New Zealand, as we shall see in Chapter 4, is different from both groups, in that there does not appear to have been an indigenous population in the sense we have used it, but the Màori settlers became their equivalent, at least in terms of their claims to the land and relations with later colonizing settlers. Ensuing history in New Zealand, however, as again we will see later, has not resulted in the degree of numerical marginalization found in the other three 'colonies', though similar oppressive processes have gone on, and the issue is far from settled (Mein Smith 2005). My impression of the *presence and relative power* of Màori people in New Zealand, however, was that it was far greater than the indigenous peoples of Australia, Canada and the USA, despite many remaining problems, and despite some moves in the other three countries at least to recognize the reality of indigenous peoples' history and to settle some land claims.

The point on colonization then also, of course, appears in the difference in the position of the monarchies of the various countries, with the European countries all having 'constitutional monarchies' while the former colonies of Australia, New Zealand and Canada still retain their technical status as subjects of the crown. The USA, as Mel Gibson (an Australian immigrant of course) has recently reminded us, became 'free' from English (and French) rule some time ago.

Table 1.1 Very brief historical comparison of the seven countries

Country	History
Sweden	Populated from Europe in pre-history. Became a consolidated kingdom in the twelfth century, which came to include Finland. Queen Margaret I of Denmark united the Nordic countries in the Kalmar Union in 1397. Continual tension within the countries and within the union gradually led to open conflict between the Swedes and the Danes in the fifteenth century. The union finally disintegrated in 1523. Involved in various European wars in sixteenth, seventeenth and eighteenth centuries. Union with Norway 1814–1905. Neutral in WWII. Constitutional monarchy and member of the EU.
Norway	Populated from Europe in pre-history. In 872, region unified under a single king. Amalgamation with Denmark and/or Sweden from 1397 as a result of Royal marriage, but also loss of Norwegian power and influence resulting from impact of Black Death. Era of short periods of both stability and unrest (see above). Independence from Sweden achieved in 1905. Occupied in WWII by 'invited' German forces. Constitutional monarchy restored after the war. Trade and other agreements with the EU, but not a member.
New Zealand	First Polynesian immigration approx 800 AD. In 1642, Dutch sailor, Tasman, visited islands but no settlement until after Cook visited over 100 years later. Formed part of the colony of New South Wales from 1788–1840. Treaty of Waitangi between Màori and Britain in 1840 created an independent constitution and crown colony. Separated (from Australia) as a dominion in 1907 and given independence 1947. Part of Allied forces in WWII. Changes to voting system from 1996 led to significant Màori presence in parliament, and Commission on Treaty of Waitangi still working on settling reclamation of lands and/or financial compensation.
Australia	Inhabited by aboriginal population for thousands of years. Claimed for England by Cook in 1770. First penal colony established in 1788. Main immigration from UK in 1850s following the discovery of gold. A series of separate colonies until the Commonwealth of Australia was established on 1 January 1901. Part of Allied forces in WWII. Referendum on constitutional change and removing the monarchy in 1999 and Senate enquiry in 2004 but no formal agreed decision for change.
Canada	Inhabited by aboriginal population for thousands of years. Viking contact around 1000 years ago with evidence of settlement. Various European contacts from fifteenth century onward. In 1608, Quebec province claimed by French though there was also a British presence in Newfoundland and other southern territories. Seven years war ended in 1763 with Treaty of Paris ceding most of the territory to Britain. In 1867 became self-governing British dominion but with significant French-speaking population and two official languages. Western provinces settled by many refugees from Europe, e.g. Ukraine, German states. Constitution of 1983 confirmed large degree of autonomy for Provinces/Territories.

USA	Inhabited by aboriginal population for thousands of years. In 1000 approx., Leif Ericson discovers NE coast. In 1493, Columbus visits offshore islands followed by various European settlers, mainly Spanish, in the south. First British settlement, Jamestown, established 1607. In 1620, Mayflower Pilgrims come from England. Declaration of Independence in 1776 followed by war between UK and the 13 eastern states forming the then union. In 1783, the Treaty of Paris gave formal separation from UK, with US Constitution written in 1789. Expansion of country westward including war with Mexico. Large influx of slaves at this time, eventually one of the causes of American Civil War, 1849–1865. Significant economic growth during late nineteenth and early twentieth centuries, with many immigrants from Europe and elsewhere. Constitutional federal government of a union of sovereign states – last to join was Hawaii.
England	Populated from Europe in pre-history. Roman occupation from 55 BC to 410 AD followed by Anglo-Saxon invasion and pushing of Celtic peoples north and west. Viking invasions in seventh to tenth centuries. Norman conquest, 1066. English (descended from Norman) King conquered Wales in 1280s and countries joined ever since (legally since 1542). Union with Scotland 1603, and formally with Ireland following the Reformation in 1689 though rebellion continued in both countries. Britain became a dominant trading and colonizing power in period of sixteenth to seventeenth centuries. Significant emigration to, especially in nineteenth century, and immigration from, especially in late twentieth century, the colonized countries. Many colonies became independent after WWII, most joining the 'British Commonwealth'. England forms part of the constitutional monarchy of the United Kingdom of Great Britain and Ireland formed by the Act of Union in 1801. The Republic of Ireland became a separate country in 1922, leaving six counties of Ulster still part of UK as Northern Ireland. Constitutional monarchy and member of the EU.

Source: Information taken from Wikipedia, the internet encyclopaedia http://en.wikipedia.org/wiki/ Main_Page accessed on various dates in November and December 2006.

What is also common to the seven countries, at least until very recent times, is the total dominance of Christianity as the religion of the majority, though of course denominational issues within Christianity were sometimes one of the causes for emigration from one country to another (Oshel.com 2007). This inevitably has a connection with welfare services but is also reflected in the debates on eugenics, sterilization, and selective screening which themselves revolve around definitions, including religious ones, of what constitutes 'humanity'. Further issues regarding populations of the different countries are raised by Table 1.2 and Figure 1.1.

Table 1.2 is taken from each country's own official statistics and so the classifications specified were those used in their own census collection. Though this raises questions of comparability, both Table 1.2 and Figure 1.1

Table 1.2 Percentages of 'ethnic' groups in the seven countries

Country	White or Caucasian	Black	Asian	Original peoples	Mixed	Other (defs differ between countries)	Source
Sweden	99.3		0.4			0.3	2005 data from http://www.scb.se/default_2154.asp# accessed 12.12.06
Norway	96.2	0.7	2.6			0.5	2001 census data from http://www.ssb.no/english/about_ssb/ accessed 12.12.06
New Zealand	70.1		6.2	8.3	7.6	8.7 (including pacific islanders)	2001 census data from http://www.stats.govt.nz/default.htm accessed 12.12.06
Australia	84.3	0.9	5.9	2.2		6.7 (including mixed and oceanic)	2001 census data from http://www.abs.gov.au/ accessed 12.12.06
Canada	64.6	2.2	7.6	3.4	21.6	1.2	2001 census data from http://www12.statcan.ca/english/census01/products accessed 12.12.06 mixed race data includes mixed Caucasian, e.g. Scottish/French mix
USA	75.1	12.3	3.6	0.9	2.4	5.6	2000 census data from http://www.census.gov/population/pop-profile/2000/chap02.pdf accessed 12.2.06 N.B. 12.5 per cent of the population categorized themselves as Hispanic as well as fitting into one of the other listed categories
UK	90.9	2.3	4.9	0	1.3	0.5	2001 census data from http://en.wikipedia.org/wiki/Demographics_of_England_from_the_2001_United_Kingdom-_census accessed 20.12.06

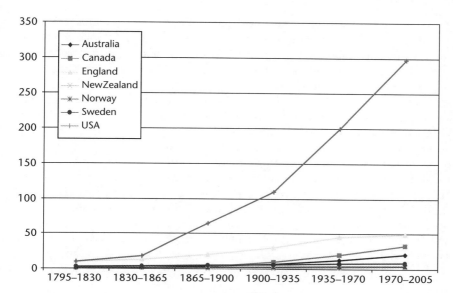

Figure 1.1 Population growth in the seven countries, 1795–2005.

support the points made on the immigrant nature of many of the countries, and the position of 'original peoples'. Table 1.2 also, of course, tells us something about the different countries' attitudes to, and recording of, data on ethnicity, something which will be explored further in individual chapters. Figure 1.1, whose order is different from the tables, in ascending size of the latest growth in population, reveals the very large rate of growth in the population of the USA beginning in the late nineteenth century and continuing to the present. This reflects the continuing immigration to that country, the imported population of the slavery years, and the second and third generations of children of immigrants and slaves then being part of the post-WWII baby boom (Internet Modern History Sourcebook 2007). All the other countries show much steadier growth rates, with Norway and Sweden virtually flat, and England increasing more strongly at the height of empire in the late nineteenth and early twentieth centuries. The 'new countries', of Australia, New Zealand, and Canada, for whom census recording only really began just before the turn of the twentieth century, also grow at a steady rate until after WWII, with New Zealand continuing to do so. The post-war period then sees the effects of a new wave of immigration to Australia, Canada and England, alongside the baby boom, and this continues in the former two countries up to date, though England levels off more recently, despite the English media's hysteria of 'alien hordes' arriving (*Daily Mail* 2005).

So growth in population, and its effects on both the culture of countries and their perceived ability to provide welfare services, have then to be considered alongside other population data. Tables 1.3 and 1.4 look at the size and density of the populations of the countries. Table 1.5 looks at urbanization, and, like Tables 1.2, 1.6 and 1.7 has an entry for the UK, rather than England. This is due to the lack of separation of English data from the rest of the UK in the source of the table.

Tables 1.3 and 1.4 reveal distinct differences between the countries, but also some grouping. Sweden, Norway and New Zealand have relatively similar geographical areas and populations, and therefore population densities, with Sweden somewhat higher than the other two. Canada and Australia, though between 20 and 40 times the areas of these other three countries, do not match this with the size of their populations, resulting in densities around 20–40 per cent of Sweden, Norway and New Zealand. The USA, on the other hand, has a similar size to Australia and Canada, in broad terms, but a population over ten times as big. So the USA has nearly twice the population density of Norway, Sweden and New Zealand, and around ten times that of Australia and Canada. The real oddity, however, is England, with the smallest land area but the second

Table 1.3   Size and population of the seven countries

Country	Land area in sq. km.	Population	Population density (people per square kilometre)
Norway	307,860	4,610,820	15.0
Sweden	410,934	9,016,596	21.9
New Zealand	268,021	4,076,140	15.2
Australia	7,617,930	20,264,082	2.7
Canada	9,093,507	33,098,932	3.6
USA	9,161,923	298,444,215	32.6
England	130,365	49,138,831	376.9

Source: Data in this and Table 1.4 are taken from the World Factbook, accessed on various dates in September and October 2006 https://www.cia.gov/cia/publications/factbook/index.html

Table 1.4   Country size, population and population density ranked with the highest first

Land area in sq. km.	Population	Population density (people per square kilometre)
USA	USA	England
Canada	England	USA
Australia	Canada	Sweden
Sweden	Australia	New Zealand
Norway	Sweden	Norway
New Zealand	Norway	Canada
England	New Zealand	Australia

Table 1.5 Urbanization levels

Country	Urban population 2003 (millions)	Percentage of total population	Average annual % growth in urban population 1990–2003	Population in urban areas of more than one million population (%)	Urban population in largest city (%)
Sweden	7.5	83	0.4	19	23
Norway	3.4	76	0.9	0*	23
New Zealand	3.5	86	1.3	28	32
Australia	18.3	92	1.8	61	23
Canada	25.1	79	1.3	37	20
USA	226.6	78	1.4	42	8
UK	53.2	90	0.3	23	14

Notes: * Oslo population approx 800,000
Urban population is the mid-year population of areas defined as urban in each country and reported to the United Nations.

Source: http://devdata.worldbank.org/wdipdfs/table3_10.pdf accessed 28.11.06

highest population. As Table 1.4 confirms, this gives England the highest population density, at over eleven times the level of the next highest country, the USA, and nearly 140 times Sweden, the country with the lowest density.

The picture becomes a little more diverse when we look at Table 1.5, showing various aspects of urbanization. Though, as might be expected from the data on England, the UK's population density gives it one of the highest proportions of urban dwelling, the country with huge areas of land and one of the lowest population densities, Australia, not only has 92 per cent of its population in urban areas, but has the fastest rate of growth in urban dwelling. UK figures also put it at the lowest of all the countries, in terms of urban population *growth*, along with the older European countries of Norway and Sweden, at a level well below 1 per cent per annum between 1990 and 2003. Once again, the relatively lower levels of immigration, at least in recent years, to these countries may be a clue to the figures, as immigrants predominantly settle in urban areas (e.g. Lind 1985; Anisef and Lanphier 2003). Despite the differences, however, *all* the countries have a high proportion of their population in urban areas, and thus can all be classed as industrialized 'Western' societies, where the sort of thinking about social and welfare policies is likely to have an urban focus (Lind 1985; Baldock et al. 2003). The spread of such a focus, in the sense of the *number* of large urban areas, which will also have an effect, as we will see, on regional variations of provision, is revealed by the figures on proportions in urban areas over one million, and in the largest city, given in Table 1.5. The particular position of Auckland in New Zealand is highlighted here, at the top end of the latter statistic, while the same column reveals the much greater number of large cities in the USA, thus making the percentage in the largest city not that great, but contributing to the figure of 42 per cent of the population being in cities of over one million. On the other hand, despite its great size geographically, Australia's urban population is concentrated in a small number of large cities, giving it the highest percentage, at 61 per cent of the population, in urban areas of more than one million.

The effects of that urbanization and industrialization may be among the reasons for the differences in populations of different ages in the countries, as well as birth rates and age expectancies, though of course other factors, especially the welfare regimes and levels of poverty, will play their part (Baldock et al. 2003). Tables 1.6 and 1.7 give data on these issues, again with England subsumed under UK figures.

Table 1.6 Population distribution of the seven countries by age

Country	0–14 (%)			15–64 (%)			65+ (%)		
	m	f	total	m	f	total	m	f	total
Sweden	8.6	8.1	**16.7**	33.3	32.4	**65.7**	7.7	10.0	**17.6**
Norway	9.9	9.4	**19.3**	33.5	32.5	**65.9**	6.3	8.6	**14.8**
New Zealand	10.8	10.3	**21.1**	33.7	33.4	**67.1**	5.2	6.6	**11.8**
Australia	10.0	9.6	**19.6**	34.0	33.4	**67.3**	5.8	7.3	**13.1**
Canada	9.0	8.6	**17.6**	34.7	34.4	**69.0**	5.7	7.6	**13.3**
USA	10.4	10.0	**20.4**	33.5	33.7	**67.2**	5.2	7.3	**12.5**
UK	9.8	9.3	**19.1**	36.9	36.1	**73.0**	7.4	9.9	**17.3**

Source: Data in this table are taken from the World Factbook accessed on various dates in September and October 2006 https://www.cia.gov/cia/publications/factbook/index.html

Table 1.7 Life expectancy and birth rates in the seven countries

Country	Life expectancy – males	Life expectancy – females	Total	Birth rate
Sweden	78.3	82.9	80.5	1.66
Norway	76.9	82.3	79.5	1.78
New Zealand	75.8	81.9	78.8	1.79
Australia	77.6	83.5	80.5	1.76
Canada	76.9	83.7	80.2	1.61
USA	75.0	80.8	77.9	2.09
UK	76.1	81.1	78.5	1.66

Source: Data in this table are taken from the World Factbook accessed on various dates in September and October 2006 https://www.cia.gov/cia/publications/factbook/index.html

There is very little to differentiate between the countries in gender terms, with only the 65+ groups varying from an approximate 50/50 gender split. Even here, the imbalance in proportions in that age category is common to all the countries, largely explained by the greater life expectancy of females. Greater variation between the countries comes, however, in the *total* proportions in the different age ranges, revealing the relatively ageing populations in the UK and Sweden, and the much younger population of New Zealand.

Life expectancies, as we have noted, contribute to a higher proportion of older people overall, but there are not major differences between the countries on this variable, except the fact that the USA, popularly seen as the most prosperous and medically advanced of all the countries, has the *lowest* life expectancy for both males and females. Given that the USA also has the highest birth rate of all the countries, this provides much food for thought on the effects of poverty at both ends of the life course, especially when connected with the lack of a comprehensive publicly funded health system in the USA (Aday 2001), and the significantly higher number of deaths through violence (Miringoff and Miringoff 1999). Issues of poverty will recur in the US chapter, as will the relation between poverty and the provision of welfare services, especially health care, a significant factor in services for people with intellectual disability. Certainly those countries with a longer history of a 'welfare state' are among the higher end of the life expectancy range, though other issues to do with lifestyle and climate also play their part, making the closeness of the figures difficult to disentangle in terms of cause and effect. More may be gleaned from Table 1.8, which looks at economic data from the different countries.

Table 1.8 confirms the place of our seven countries in the group of nations, with relatively high wealth and low unemployment, that have dominated the world economic system for over a century, though now facing significant impacts from the emerging economies of the highly populated countries of India and China. None of these countries could therefore be described as poor, but the most recent experiences of relative poverty, found in the 1930s in Sweden and Norway, are said by many to have contributed significantly to the establishment of their welfare states (Kautto et al. 1999). It is also said to have contributed to a still existing lower variation in income and wealth distribution, to some extent borne out in Table 1.8. with Norway and Sweden having the highest percentage of people receiving the top 10 per cent of national income, and the lowest percentage receiving the bottom 10 per cent, revealing the flatter distribution of income in those two countries. The period of neo-liberal economics, begun in the 1980s in the USA and the UK with the Thatcher/Reagan eras, and continuing to dominate the global economy, can also be observed in terms of the other countries' performance on this income distribution data. The lowest proportion of people receiving the top 10 per cent of income, and the highest proportion receiving the bottom 10 per cent are found, unsurprisingly, in the USA, closely followed by the UK and Australia. Canada is

Table 1.8   Selected economic and social welfare statistics for the seven countries

Country	GDP (ppp*) per capita in $	Unemployment (%)	National income received by the bottom 10% of households in the income distribution (%)	National income received by the top 10% of households in the income distribution (%)	Public debt as a % of GDP	% of GDP spent on welfare
Sweden	29,800	5.8	3.7	20.1	50.4	28.9
Norway	42,300	4.6	4.1	21.8	50.1	23.9
New Zealand	25,200	3.7	NA	NA	21.3	18.5
Australia	31,900	5.1	2.0	25.4	16.1	18.0
Canada	34,000	6.8	2.8	23.8	69.6	17,8
USA	41,800	5.1	1.8	30.5	64.7	14.8
UK	30,300	4.7	2.1	28.5	43.1	21.8

Note: * PPP stands for purchasing power parity. The PPP method of assessing Gross Domestic product involves the use of standardized international dollar price weights, which are applied to the quantities of final goods and services produced in a given economy. The data derived from the PPP method probably provide the best available starting point for comparisons of economic strength and well-being between countries.

Source: Data in this table are taken from the World Factbook accessed on various dates in September and October 2006 https://www.cia.gov/cia/publications/factbook/index.html

then in between this group and the Scandinavians, with, frustratingly, no available data from this source for New Zealand. Such a distribution of the nations' wealth does not, however, appear to be correlated with the size of that wealth, since oil-rich Norway still seems to have managed to keep its wealth distribution fairly flat, despite having the highest per capita GDP, and Sweden does the same with the second lowest per capita GDP. The same goes for public debt and welfare spending, with the countries with highest level of debt, the USA and Canada, having the lowest level of welfare spending. Sweden comes highest in the proportion of GDP spent on welfare, nearly twice that of the USA, and there does appear to be a connection, which would be expected, between the degree of comprehensiveness of the welfare state in the different countries and the proportion of their GDP spent on welfare. This connection does not appear, however, as we have noted, to exist between the *size* of GDP and the proportion spent on welfare, nor between the proportion spent on welfare and the level of unemployment. Canada has the highest level of unemployment, but the second lowest proportion of GDP spent on welfare, while Sweden's highest level of welfare spending goes along with the second highest unemployment rate. Instead, this latter data suggest that government policies on payments to the unemployed, including of course large numbers of people with intellectual disabilities, and on free or subsidized healthcare, are much more influential in determining levels of expenditure (Alcock and Craig 2001).

We end this demographic overview with a look at how the countries compare on the UN Human Development Index (HDI) (United Nations 2006). This comparative measure of poverty, literacy, education, life expectancy, child birth, and other factors is a standard means of measuring well-being for countries worldwide. Developed in 1990 by Pakistani economist Mahbub ul Haq, it has been used since 1993 by the United Nations Development Programme in its annual Human Development Report. The HDI measures the average achievements in a country in three basic dimensions of human development:

- a long and healthy life, as measured by life expectancy at birth;
- knowledge, as measured by the adult literacy rate (with two-thirds weight) and the combined primary, secondary, and tertiary education gross enrollment ratio (with one-third weight);
- a decent standard of living, as measured by gross domestic product (GDP) per capita at purchasing power parity (PPP) in US dollars.

Figure 1.2 shows the ranking, in relation to the scores of all the countries in the United Nations, of our seven countries, and immediately confirms all of them to be among the highest scoring, with every one in the top twenty world ranking.

Some of our previous statistics may give a clue to the relative positions of the different countries, with the differential weighting given to the elements of the HDI being a key element. They will lead us to expect that the high GDP, therefore, of Norway, combined with its relatively high birth rate, would put it among the leaders, and when we add in the education policies that we will discuss in Chapter 3, it comes as no surprise that Norway is at number one.

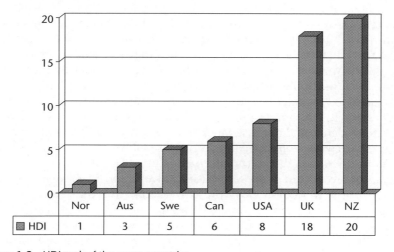

	Nor	Aus	Swe	Can	USA	UK	NZ
HDI	1	3	5	6	8	18	20

Figure 1.2 HDI rank of the seven countries.

The fairly similar, and high, life expectancy of Australia, Canada, and Sweden then also combines with their above average GDP to place them in the position to have a high ranking, with the literacy and education variables, I would surmise, also maintaining that level. The last two variables of the index would be my guess as to why the USA, despite its high GDP, is in eighth place. We have seen how its life expectancy is lower than the others, and will see in Chapter 6 how the huge variation between States in terms of education, combined with a much lower literacy rate among a significant number of poor and immigrant people, would lead to a low score on the second element of the HDI. As for the UK, while its life expectancy levels are still high by world standards, we saw in Table 1.7 that it was still the second lowest of the seven countries. When this is combined with a middle range GDP, but especially taking account of the UK's still relatively low literacy levels and its school-leaving age, for the majority, of 16, as compared with 18–20 for the majority of the other countries, its ranking is not surprising. The only surprise to me in the HDI ranking was New Zealand, although, as we have already noted, it is still twentieth in the world. A possible reason could be found in its GDP level, which as Table 1.8 shows, is significantly lower than the other six countries. The life expectancy, possibly disproportionately affected by crime and poverty among the Màori and Pacific Island peoples (Durie 2005), is also one of the lowest, and despite many efforts, issues of literacy and education, and how they are defined, are also tied up with the ethnic mix of the young country.

Conclusion – a world tour of seven affluent countries

The final set of data of this chapter is, for me, the most sobering, when it comes to writing the rest of the book. In terms of the subtle differences between seven countries, all in the top twenty on the UN HDI, we can already begin to see issues that will be teased out as we go through the individual chapters. We can also see, however, why readers from other countries, especially those significantly lower down the HDI scale, might find those subtleties fairly meaningless, compared to their basic struggles to obtain any sort of standard of life, or even life itself. It is not an original thought, but one which I have repeated often to students, and to those I met on my study leave, that looking at how societies deal with people with intellectual disabilities reveals the more general cracks in the façade of civilization that we in the comfortable 'top twenty' put forward to the rest of the world. Paradoxically, too, I believe how we treat the rest of the world, especially those 'we' regard as significantly 'different' from 'us' in, to use a phrase from SRV, behaviour, appearance or social functioning, is reflected in how we treat those in our own country with intellectual disabilities. It is not for nothing that the English called their institutions in the first half of the twentieth century 'colonies'.

2　Sweden

Rational, orderly, enjoyable and healthy lives?

At last the Dodo said, 'Everybody has won, and all must have prizes.'

(Lewis Carroll)

INSTANT IMPACTS

Sweden – an unknown housemate

As a guest of the University of Jonkoping, I was housed in an apartment near the campus, on the second floor of a four-storey block, one of three round a grassed courtyard. On my second morning, as I was leaving for the walk to the university, I passed the door of a first floor apartment as it opened. As I reached the ground floor, I could hear somebody saying what I guessed to be the Swedish for 'good-bye and have a good day' and as I exited the communal front door of the block, I could see coming down the stairs a woman with Down's syndrome, probably in her thirties. She clearly knew the exit routes from the complex better than I did, for when I emerged on to the busy main road to the university, the woman had already come out, ahead of me, via another exit. I was able to observe, therefore, how she proceeded to cross the main road and disappear down another street. I discovered, in the course of my time in Sweden, that this was not a remarkable occurrence. The Swedish law gives entitlement to people with intellectual disabilities to their own apartments, subsidized to some extent, but also affordable by their fairly substantial benefits. Such is one of the results of their implementation of 'normalization' over the nearly 40 years since Bengt Nirje and Karl Grunewald, among others, articulated the aims of their service system in those terms.

Introduction – return to a welfare state

In 1976, as young research workers, my wife and I visited services in Sweden. The man organizing our trip was Karl Grunewald, then known as a key figure, along with Niels Bank-Mikkelsen from Denmark, Wolf Wolfensberger from the USA, and Bengt Nirje, also from Sweden, in the small group of people promulgating the set of ideas called 'normalization' (Nirje 1999; Wolfensberger 1999). What we found in Sweden (Race and Race 1978), was something of a contrast, even to the 'radical' project with which we were involved, itself very different to many UK services. The contrast was not only in the 'model' of services, which particularly manifested itself in the community-based residential developments then beginning in Sweden, but also in the organizational and governance arrangements for services. We knew, of course, of the 'model welfare state' reputation of Sweden but it was the fact that one 'state' service existed for people with intellectual disabilities, run at 'county' level, that gave us the sharpest difference with the UK, with its twin state service bodies of the National Health Service and Local Authority (LA hereafter) Social Services Departments. Returning 29 years later, with all the changes that had taken place in my own country, the main contrast that hit me was that Sweden had retained, to a large extent, its welfare state, despite what was going on in the rest of the world, but that it had also now devolved services to a more local level. What I observed in 2005 was a national policy, in the form of the various laws governing entitlements to services, but local responsibility for implementation.

Without wishing to labour the point, the importance of Swedish intellectual disability services existing within a system of state *funding*, via taxation, *and* state *provision* of services, with workers in the field being mostly local authority (usually translated as 'municipality') employees, or, if not, employees of the county health service, needs to be strongly emphasized. Sweden and Norway are the only countries that have this overwhelming domination of the service system by local and national government, controlling funding *as well as* employing and managing those involved in the direct provision of services. As another English observer of social policy in Sweden put it, 'through the welfare state, among other institutions, Sweden has sought to create a rational stable society in which the vast majority of its people can lead rational, orderly, enjoyable and healthy lives' (Gould 2001: 192). This raises the question, for our purposes, as to how far Swedish society has included in that 'vast majority' people with intellectual disabilities and their families. To begin to answer that question we must examine the history of services for people with an intellectual disability in Sweden.

Historical development of services – from segregation to normalization and beyond

Early developments – Sweden as part of Europe

It is perhaps a truism to state that the history of European services for people with intellectual disabilities is related to the history of how intellectual impairment has been viewed by European societies. It also follows that developments in intellectual disability services relate to notions of welfare in general, and the role of the state in this, and how the very issue of a state role emerged most sharply as urbanization and industrialization took hold in Europe in the nineteenth century (Baldock et al. 2003). What of Sweden? Kent Ericsson takes up the story, with issues that will be echoed in later chapters:

> The residential institution, as a way of delivering support from society to persons with a disability, grew out of the conditions in the second half of the 19th century. This was a period of change in Sweden when an old agrarian society was transformed into an industrial society. During this change persons with a disability became 'visible', a group among others. The families of these persons turned to society for assistance but there were few public services at that time to respond to the needs they expressed. A natural consequence was that private organizations for assistance were created. Later on public bodies also began to form disability services. The support of this period was delivered through residential institutions, where a group was taken care of, often in the countryside. Education was arranged for the 'educable', care for the 'uneducable'.
>
> During the 19th century work was carried out with optimism, and an ambition that persons would return to those communities from which they had originally come. But the eugenics of the first half of the 20th century gave new conditions for disability services. A more protective attitude created walls, physically and metaphorically, around the residential institutions. They became places where large groups were kept under poor conditions.
>
> (Ericsson 2000: 3)

Mention of 'the eugenics of the first half of the 20th century' not only brings developments in Sweden once again into line with events in Europe, but also the USA and the 'colonies' of the British Empire, such as Canada, Australia and New Zealand. When talking about 'views of society', of people with intellectual disabilities, those latter countries had the extra issues of views about the 'civilization' of the indigenous populations and their subsequent treatment by the colonizers. In addition, in the USA, there was the impact of more than two centuries of imported slaves and its boiling point in the Civil War. Details of these latter countries will be given in their respective chapters, but it is important to spend extra time, in this first chapter bearing on history, in noting how widespread notions of 'racial superiority' engendered by the colonization and slave trading of many countries in the eighteenth, and especially the nineteenth, centuries, combined with and exacerbated growing ideas of the 'inheritance of defect', known more commonly now as the 'eugenics movement' (Race 2002b).

Eugenics – Sweden as part of the 'civilized world'

In these days of mass education and widespread communication, it can be difficult to understand the undoubted fact that a relatively small, but highly powerful, group of academics, politicians and policy-makers were able to influence, and radically change, the form and content of what was provided to people with intellectual disabilities in the first half of the twentieth century. This was especially true of Northern Europe, with the venerable, and vener- ated, post-Enlightenment university tradition of 'reason and rationality' creat- ing what amounted to a consensus on both 'inheritance of defect' and the 'worthlessness' of individuals in utilitarian terms. The views of the English leader in this field, Tredgold, sum up what was a widely held view in these intellectual elites

> as soon as a nation reaches that stage of civilisation in which medical knowledge and humanitarian sentiment operate to prolong the exist- ence of the unfit, then it becomes imperative upon that nation to devise such social laws as will ensure that those unfit do not propagate their kind.
>
> (Tredgold 1909: 8)

The hope, as Ericsson reminds us above, of the 'trainability' of people from the nineteenth-century institutions, meaning their eventual return home, was thus replaced by what amounted to an ideolology of segregation, but one given significant credibility by the support of 'scientific and medical' research. The idea of an inherited intellectual ability, which is unaltered by training or education, and in fact determines one's response to education or training, was not new at the turn of the century, but was somewhat in a minority. The combination, however, of genetic 'findings' on the inherit- ability of many characteristics, beyond physiological ones such as eye colour, and the arrival of a supposedly 'scientific measure' of intelligence persuaded many in academic circles of the invariance of this 'inherent ability' (Gould 1996; Race 2002a). Reaction from the eugenics movement is again graphically laid out by Tredgold, but with an order of priority that was to have particular implications beyond the institutions that followed in many countries, including Sweden.

> 1. In the first place the chief evil we have to prevent is undoubtedly that of propagation. 2. Next, society must be protected against such of these persons as either have definite criminal tendencies, or are of so facile a disposition that they readily commit crimes at the instigation of others. 3. Lastly, even where these poor creatures are relatively harmless, we have to protect society from the burden due to their non-productiveness.
>
> (Tredgold 1909: 3)

The institutions that then burgeoned around Europe could carry out Tredgold's second point fairly easily, and by putting the more able to work for the institution, they could go a long way towards the third. As for the first point, however, merely incarcerating individuals did not seem to be enough. Sterilization, backed by law in many places, became overt policy in almost all institutions (Broberg and Roll-Hansen 2005) and was then applied, in some countries, to people with intellectual disabilities *not* in institutions, often with the support of parents.

Given the widespread nature of the eugenic view in the period between the wars, it is, therefore, perhaps ironic that 'revelations' from an academic thesis by Maija Runcis, an archivist working for the Swedish government, published in 1998 (Runcis 1998), but whose contents had been taken up by the media in 1997, should have caused enough of a stir for the Swedish Minister for Social Affairs to apologize to the nation and seek to reimburse 'victims' of the Swedish sterilization law.

Perhaps the 'severe embarrassment' to the government in 1997 was more to its reputation outside Sweden, as the 'model' welfare state, especially when it came to intellectual disability, or perhaps it stemmed from the association with the Nazi regime's taking of eugenics to its logical conclusion, and actually killing large numbers of people in the *euthanasie* programme of the late 1930s, in what some saw as a rehearsal for the Holocaust (Lifton 1986). Whatever the reason, the law had continued up to 1975, the year before my first visit to Sweden, resulting in the reported sterilization of some 63,000 people over the previous 40 years, without seemingly affecting Sweden's reputation for progressive services, the very reason for that visit. I cannot recall it being mentioned all those years ago, and, on the recent visit, the existence still of a process for sterilization with parental consent was discussed by parents in a matter-of-fact way.

The impression, therefore, of the situation up to World War II in Sweden is one of the growing importance of the state, via the social democratic ideal but also via the weight given to 'scientific knowledge', in determining what was in the best interests of society. The consensus of that scientific knowledge therefore meant that people with intellectual disabilities were the recipients of services designed to keep them safe, and to keep society safe from them. Gynnerstedt (1997) defines this as the period of clientalism. 'The issues of independence, integrity and privacy for the clients were non-existent. Those with learning disabilities were looked upon as clients/patients and the expected behaviours were passive, accepting, patient and grateful' (ibid.: 149).

Normalization – Swedish and Scandinavian roots

Readers from other countries will, I would suggest, be familiar with the above description of institutional thinking, and may then ask how the next 25 years or so saw Sweden become the model for visiting scholars in the field. Many writers (e.g. Kristiansen et al. 1999) point to two significant factors. First, the influence of leaders and pressure groups from outside the traditional 'expert' bodies, especially the parents' group FUB (the Swedish acronym for the body translated into English as 'the Swedish National Association for persons and adults with mental handicap'). Second, in the 1960s, the ratification in policy of an already existing but previously under-utilized commitment that the 'patterns of life' available to all citizens be made available to those with disabilities. As Ericsson (2000) points out, the notion of 'normalization of citizenship' had existed in written form in Sweden as far back as 1946, when a committee, set up to propose how the 'partially able-bodied', an interestingly modern-sounding translation from the Swedish *partiellt arbetsfora*, would be part of the post-war welfare state, included in their report the following

> this, even for the partially able-bodied themselves, must be seen as a basic right as a citizen; it is entirely in keeping with the very essence of democracy that equal human value and equal rights are put in the foreground ... Psychologically this 'normalisation' of conditions of life, education, employment exchange etc. of the partially able-bodied must be a great achievement.
>
> (SOU 1946: 24: 28)

The real point of this quotation is not to enter the rather esoteric sport of spotting the first use of the word 'normalization' but to highlight the committee's notion of the 'basic right as a citizen', based on 'equal human value and equal rights'. Though only adopted in limited fashion immediately after the war, the root of the idea was to emerge in the development of what Nirje and others were to call 'the normalization principle' in the 1960s. In Nirje's (1999) view, however, moves towards the goal of normalization had begun before its widespread publication in the late 1960s, and here we return to the first of the two factors for change – the emergence of national leaders and the influence of

FUB. Nirje himself, of course, is one of those leaders, and provides the link with FUB. Nirje had been appointed in 1961 as 'ombudsman' for FUB, then five years old as a national organization. At that point, 'professional' services consisted almost entirely of residential schools, under the aegis of the Swedish Board of Education, and the large institutions, under the Royal Medical Board. FUB, perhaps seeing actions by parents groups elsewhere, were intending to set up a service-providing organization. They also saw an increase in local associations from 55 to over 100, and were active in trying to persuade the government to bring in new legislation, with alternatives to institutional provision. Like parents around the world, however, FUB members differed greatly in what they saw as suitable services for their 'children' of whatever age. Many were totally happy to take the professional view that 'expertise' was to be found in the institutions; many became ardent supporters of institutions; and many were, quite simply, grateful for services of any kind, having often had nothing. Nirje (1999: 24) notes that even the sub-committees within FUB, set up to try and put forward draft legislation around alternatives to institutions, were 'cautious, apprehensive and dissatisfied' though whether the last feeling was with existing conditions or the new proposals he does not say.

It was at this time that the international group that was to become influential in the spreading of normalization began to make contact, and they had perhaps their most influential period at the end of the 1960s with the publication, including contributions from nearly all the key figures, of a report for the US President's Committee, edited and organized largely by Wolfensberger, that was later published as *Changing Patterns in Residential Services for the Mentally Retarded* (Kugel and Wolfensberger 1969). As the personal accounts of both Wolfensberger (1999) and Nirje (1999) attest, this much referred to but less often read publication had a very haphazard, not to say almost farcical nascence, and might have merely gathered dust on bureaucratic shelves, had it not coincided with a mood of change in those countries from where the leaders came, especially Sweden, with Nirje and Grunewald, Denmark, with Bank-Mikkelsen and North America, with Wolfensberger and Dybwad. It also contained the first written account of the 'normalization principle' written by Nirje in his chapter of the same name.

The Swedish contribution to these movements was made all the more credible by the formulation, in 1967, of a new Act for Services to the Mentally Retarded. Though this represented a significant advance on the sole provision of institutions, and incorporated into state provision many of the community-based services previously started by groups such as FUB, it would not be until a later piece of legislation, in 1986, that *all* people with intellectual disabilities had the legal right to participate in community life. Nevertheless the tone of the 1968 legislation and the activities of the international network certainly contributed to the reputation of Sweden as being, by the early 1970s, at the 'leading edge' of services.

By 1976, when my wife and I visited, that was still the case, though events in North America had possibly shifted the locus of dynamic change to the other side of the Atlantic. The international network at the heart of *Changing Patterns* had been, to a lesser extent, also involved in the putting together by Wolfensberger of *Normalization: The Principle of Normalization in Human Services* (Wolfensberger 1972), in which Nirje wrote a chapter entitled 'The Right to Self-Determination'. With hindsight he saw this as the beginnings of a difference in the use and articulation of the ideas between Sweden and North America, or at least between Nirje and Wolfensberger (Nirje 1999). Ideas of self-determination also seem to have caused some ripples in the 'leading edge' services in Sweden, as the full effects of the 1968 law played themselves out in practice. Gynnerstedt (1997), in calling the period from this point up to the 1980s 'welfarism', seems to imply a smooth connection between rights being prescribed by law and people being fully participating citizens, including involvement in decision-making. Nirje's chapter heading referred to above also implies that such involvement follows from the normalization principle, yet he writes (Nirje 1999: 40) of being treated as a 'danger to the intellectually disabled' by encouraging people to be so involved. Ericsson (1999) perhaps catches the picture with greater subtlety, when he talks of 'two traditions' operating at the same time. One, the 'institutional tradition' with its emphasis on education and care, on remedying a 'deficit', means the need for specialist places, specialist professionals, and the attribution of the 'client' or 'pupil' roles to people. This stands in contrast to the 'community tradition' where people are attributed the roles of citizen, with entitlements to services and opportunities afforded to all citizens, including involvement in decisions that affect their lives.

De-institutionalization – attitudes as well as buildings?

These opinions suggest, for me, the slight differences between developments in Sweden and the other countries. Those who have read Wolfensberger's work after the publication of *Normalization*, e.g. (Wolfensberger and Glenn 1975; Wolfensberger and Thomas 1983), but even the 1972 document itself, will be in no doubt as to the intrinsic part that integration holds in both his version of normalization and in its successor, SRV. If, on the other hand, we review Nirje's statement of the 'normalization principle' that remained in use in Sweden for many years (and could still be said to be the basis of services today), the issue of integration is not really addressed. The 1993 formulation that Nirje cited in Ottawa in 1994 is the clearest concise statement of the principle as used in Sweden.

> The Normalization principle means that you act right when you make available to all persons with intellectual or other impairments or

disabilities those patterns of life and conditions of everyday living that are as close as possible to, or indeed the same as, the regular circumstances and ways of life of their communities and their culture . . .

1. A normal rhythm of the day.
2. A normal rhythm of the week.
3. A normal rhythm of the year.
4. The normal experiences of the life cycle.
5. Normal respect for the individual and the right to self-determination.
6. The normal sexual patterns of their culture.
7. The normal economic patterns and rights of their society.
8. The normal environment patterns and standards in their community.

The proper use of the Normalization principle rests on an understanding of how the normal rhythms, routines, and patterns of life in any culture relate to the development, maturity, and life of disabled persons. It also rests on an understanding of how these patterns apply as indicators of *proper* human programs, services, and legislation.

(Nirje 1999: 17, emphasis in original)

As we go through the impressions of services in Sweden in 2006, the phrase *'proper* human programs, services, and legislation' could well be the way in which these could be summarized. What is less certain, as later writers such as Ericsson (2000), Gynnerstedt (1997), and Tideman (2005) point out, is whether that summary equates to community participation, or what Wolfensberger, as far back as 1972, called 'social integration'. Certainly, the period between the two pieces of legislation of 1986 and 1994 seems to have been one of important change, as the 1986 law's acknowledgement, noted above, that *all* people could live outside institutions, created first alarm and then expectations from the still powerful parents' lobby, as they saw people in the new apartments and group homes, living in ordinary communities. Those writers cited above have more doubts, however, about whether services had got very far beyond *physical* integration, and into *social* integration, and, beyond this, whether even social integration, as defined by normalization, went far enough in allowing people to exercise a degree of control and 'self-determination' in their lives (Hollander 1999).

On the ground, the large institutions were closing, with people moving to apartments and other small shared living arrangements, all specified by the 1986 law, along with the beginnings of moves towards work-based occupation in real work settings rather than segregated workshops. For children, moves away from segregated special schools towards inclusion in regular schools were also beginning, in line with international movements in this area (Booth and

Ainscow 1998). Research on the moves away from the institutions was largely positive (Ericsson 2000), in the sense that people and their families expressed no desire to go back to the institutions, though again the issues of full community participation and self-determination were the greatest causes of concern. Still more legislative change was therefore felt to be necessary, with Grunewald still playing a significant leadership role, and in 1994 the wide-ranging 'Act Concerning Support and Service for Persons with Certain Functional Impairments' (known by the abbreviated initials, LSS, of its full name in Swedish – *Lag om stod och service for vissa funktionshindrade*) came into force. Along with LSS came the reversion, for the first time, of intellectual disability services to the municipalities, except for health services, which were to remain the responsibilities of the county councils. This did not mean, however, that a 'rival' set of services existed at county level, with the complications of professional and financial allocations being based on different bureaucratic loyalties and systems, such as still bedevils services in the UK (Glasby and Peck 2004). LSS is very clear that the responsibility of county health services, which are generic health services available to all, is a limited part of its requirements, mainly in the early years, whereas the bulk of specialist services rest with the municipalities, along with their generic responsibilities for public housing, education, and other social services. Education Acts, up to and including the current one (http://www.sweden.gov.se/sb/d/2098/a/67912) have also stressed the rights to equal access to education for all children, and, following the pattern of LSS, education for children with intellectual disabilities passed in 1996 from county councils to the municipalities. Finally, as the definite culmination of the 'de-institutionalization' period, the Abolition of Institutions Act of 1997 set the final closure date, perhaps symbolically, of all institutions as 31 December 1999. Data from the survey by Mansell et al. of institutions in Europe, published in 2004, claims that Sweden is one of the few countries to have succeeded in 'de-institutionalization', at least as far as removing segregated physical buildings and 'integrating people into society' is concerned. In the rest of this chapter we will look in some detail at what this means at the different stages, from 'pre-birth to death' for people with intellectual disabilities in Sweden.

Services in Sweden – an impression

What counts as services?

As the Introduction to this book noted, the quest for what happens in the lives of people with intellectual disabilities in the different countries was structured around formal services, but looked to go beyond these to try and get a sense of what other influences were important in each country to the well-being or otherwise of this group of people. In later chapters this will take us into some interesting matters of definition, and in each chapter the significance of the different roles played by parents in the various countries will be highlighted. It is therefore not always going to be possible to look at 'services' in a neat organizational form, and so the overview which follows in Table 2.1, whose format will be repeated in the other chapters, contains very broad headings. The details which follow in each chapter are then intended to put that overview into an organizational, financial, and governance context, though because of their transitory nature, actual figures of spending on services or of benefit levels will not be given, except to compare similar services within countries.

Bearing in mind the LSS law which dictates much of Swedish services, but as a supplement to basic generic services to all citizens, Table 2.1 provides the aforementioned summary.

Table 2.1 Schematic overview of 'services' that affect the lives of people with intellectual disabilities in Sweden

'Service'	Formal organizational place	Specialist or generic?	Main source(s) of funding
Pre-natal services	County health services – Clinics and Habilitation teams	Generic and specialist	Taxation, raised by counties and 'equalized' by central government
Post-natal and early childhood services	County health services – Habilitation teams Municipal early childhood services	Generic, but with input dependent on individual children	Taxation, raised by counties and municipalities and 'equalized' by central government
Non-educational services for children	Municipal services	Specialist	Taxation, raised by municipalities and 'equalized' by central government – also National Social Insurance payments for personal assistance
Education services – children and young adults	Municipal services	Generic and specialist	Taxation, raised by municipalities and 'equalized' by central government

(Continued overleaf)

Table 2.1 Continued.

'Service'	Formal organizational place	Specialist or generic?	Main source(s) of funding
Education services – adults	Central government for universities and colleges Swedish Agency for Flexible Learning	Generic and specialist	Taxation, raised by municipalities and 'equalized' by central government
Residential services – adults	Municipal services	Generic and specialist	Taxation, raised by municipalities and 'equalized' by central government
Daytime services – non-work	Municipal services	Largely specialist	Taxation, raised by municipalities and 'equalized' by central government
Daytime services – work	Municipal services	Largely specialist	Taxation, raised by municipalities and 'equalized' by central government
Leisure assistance	Municipal services, FUB	Largely specialist	Taxation, raised by municipalities and 'equalized' by central government
Advocacy services	Municipal services – but 'good man' not employed by municipality	Specialist	Taxation, raised by municipalities and 'equalized' by central government
Financial Assistance	Swedish National Social Insurance Board	Specialist within generic service	Taxation, distributed to Social Insurance Board by central government
Parental 'support services'	Acting as all parents – not a job in an organization, but can be active in FUB	Specialist, in that all children are different	Own finances, plus some grants via municipalities or Social Insurance Board

What then follows is more detail of the elements, from the literature and from impressions gained during my visits to, or discussions about, each of them. We begin with the situation before birth.

Pre-natal services – bucking the Western trend?

In the history section above, we noted the 'embarrassment' caused to the Swedish welfare system by the 'revelations' about what had actually been a totally legal and accepted practice of sterilization of people with intellectual disabilities. This may go some way to explaining why the Swedish pre-natal system, especially in terms of screening of disabled children, differs, in my view, from most of the industrialized world, in terms of its emphasis being generally in favour of their birth. As we shall see in later chapters, identification and 'screening out' of babies with disabilities are not only common in most of the other countries (though Norway is similar to Sweden in this regard) but the promotion of such 'screening out' is sometimes the subject of specific government policy or the expectations of legal precedent.

The sterilization issue may also explain my own pre-conceptions (with apologies for the possible pun) of how Sweden dealt with the issue of abortion and pre-natal screening. A 'rational and clinical' approach would sum up these views, and, in one sense, this was borne out in my discussions with social workers in the general county hospital who counselled parents on abortion and sterilization issues.

Their job was to counsel those mothers who wished to have an abortion, available on demand under Swedish law up to 18 weeks, and those who sought or were offered screening. So far, so 'rational and clinical'; in another sense, however, their surprise on hearing that my son was adopted, effectively from birth, gave a clue as to the general emphasis of the health system in Sweden, and the positive role of 'habilitation teams', multi-disciplinary professional groups called in before the birth of a disabled child, if this is known. The social workers were unaware of any disabled children given up for adoption at birth, a view borne out by the literature, e.g. Hessle and Vinnerljung (1999), and also informed me that, as again confirmed by others, 'No policy for pre-natal screening of Down's syndrome exists in Sweden' (Annerén and Ollars 2004: 21). (NB: where direct quotations or official titles in the different countries are concerned, we will use the terminology of the country. Otherwise 'Down's syndrome' will be the term used for this condition.)

Discussion with social workers actually from the 'habilitation team', again at the county hospital, gave more details of the role of these teams. If an abnormality in pregnancy is discovered, then a second opinion is sought to confirm the result. If a specific condition is then identified, a paediatrician is called in to explain to the parents possible futures, as well as their receiving input from the various professionals in the habilitation team as appropriate. This then continues after the birth of the child.

This is not to suggest that no abortion takes place for reasons of disability, but more that the direction and source of 'pressure' seem to come from a choice being placed with the parents without, as in other countries, an implied expectation of what that choice 'should be'. What might be called 'routine' pre-natal diagnosis of Down's syndrome is based on offering amniocentesis to women 35 years of age or older and those with a significant family history of disability. This is the general view of Swedish practice, though in some places (including the hospital I visited) the practice for *all* parents who are worried about having a child with Down's syndrome is similar to that operating more generally for women *younger* than 35 years of age. This is that they are offered the pre-natal diagnosis tests, and the costs are fully reimbursed, but the first move is made by the parents. According to Annerén and Ollars (2004), half of all pregnant women who are offered pre-natal diagnosis take up the offer. In discussion, the norm where I visited was for mothers to be offered tests at their request, and usually those who requested tests opted for an abortion if an abnormality was found. Some mothers over 35, on the other hand, would not take the 'routine' test for Down's syndrome if they knew they would continue with the pregnancy regardless.

Early childhood services – habilitation and early intervention

We have noted the significant place that habilitation teams play in the time surrounding the birth of a child with obvious intellectual disabilities. Where the intellectual disability is less clear, it tends to be in the early years, through the assessment of professionals such as early childhood specialists from the municipality, that the need for extra support becomes identified. Most children, intellectually disabled or not, will have received visits from the generic child health and social care professionals in their early years, and calls on the habilitation teams will often stem from these visits. Once intellectual disability is established, however, the full range of professionals that make up the habilitation team will tend to become involved, and this is the usual way in which the need for assistance through LSS is ascertained. Support through LSS has to be applied for by parents themselves, and is subject to the decision of the locally based LSS handling officer (*LSS-handlaggere*). Habilitation teams will often help in this process, and it is again more straightforward in the obvious cases of learning disability such as Down's syndrome, whereas parents whose child is less clearly intellectually disabled may have more difficulty in accessing LSS. The formal definitions under which the LSS officer will work are summarized below, from the official government body that oversees policy, known as *Socialstyrelsen*.

The LSS applies to:

1. persons with an intellectual disability, autism or a condition resembling autism;
2. persons with a significant and permanent intellectual impairment after brain damage in adulthood due to an external force or a physical illness;
3. persons who have other major and permanent physical or mental impairments which are clearly not due to normal ageing and which cause considerable difficulties in daily life and consequently an extensive need of support and service.

(Socialstyrelsen 2006: 1)

The possibility then exists for parents to access both generic daytime child care facilities, and those that are more specialist, usually for children with severe needs. As the child grows older, LSS can then provide other services.

Non-educational services for children

The following aspects of LSS apply to both early childhood and then later on, with some specifically for certain age groups. We will quote the details (and the numbering from the ten specific headings in LSS) from the *Socialstyrelsen* summary noted above.

1 *Counselling and other personal support* – The rights to qualified expert help from staff who, in addition to their professional skills, have special knowledge of what it is like to live with major functional impairment(s) . . . Counselling and support are to be a supplement to, and not a replacement for measures such as habilitation, rehabilitation and social welfare services.

2 *Personal assistance* – Persons with major functional impairments and an extensive need of support and help in their daily lives may be entitled to personal assistance from one or more personal assistants. The municipality is financially responsible for those who need assistance for less than 20 hours a week.

   If a person needs personal assistance for their basic needs for more than 20 hours a week, they may be entitled to assistance benefit. The right to this benefit is set out in LASS – the Assistance Benefit Act (1993: 389).

3 *Companion service* – Those not entitled to personal assistance may instead be entitled to a companion service. The companion service is to be a personal service, adapted to individual needs, designed to make it easier for the individual to participate in the life of the community.

4   *Personal contact* – A personal contact is to be a companion who can help the individual to lead an independent life by reducing social isolation, helping them take part in recreational activities and providing advice in everyday situations. This support can sometimes be provided by a family, known as a support family.

5   *Relief service in the home* – A relief service can be provided on a regular basis as well as for unexpected situations. It is to be available round the clock.

6   *Short stay away from the home* – Short stays away from the home are to provide the individual with recreation and a change of scene, while giving relatives a break. A short-term stay can be in a respite home, in another family or in another way, e.g. a stay at a youth camp or holiday camp.

7   *Short period of supervision for schoolchildren over the age of 12* Schoolchildren over the age of 12, who are no longer covered by general childcare services, can receive supervision before and after the school day and during school holidays.

8   *Living in family homes or homes with special service for children and young persons* – Children and young persons who cannot live with their parents may be entitled to live with another family or in a home with special service. This is to be a supplement to the parental home, both for children who can live with their parents some of the time, and for those who cannot live with their parents at all.

(Socialstyrelsen 2006: 1–2)

This, of course is the official picture, and we shall see that such presentations of 'available services' in other countries are not always matched by the reality. As a legal 'right', however, the culture of Swedish society, plus the ability to appeal to a County Administrative Court, does appear to ensure a large degree of compliance. Since the municipalities have to implement the legislation via their normal budget, however, as well as finance generic services for their local inhabitants, this does cause tension between the national and local levels of government, with a few municipalities defying the courts.

Overall, however, the picture for intellectually disabled children in Sweden, in terms of non-educational services, is a fairly positive one. It will be noted that eight out of the ten requirements under LSS apply to children, though some carry through to adulthood, but it is through early intervention, in my view, that a more positive view of support, then backed up by that support itself, is provided. Hence my summary of Adam's chances if he were in Sweden (see box).

ADAM'S WORLD TOUR

Conceived in Sweden – what next?

If Adam were conceived in Sweden now, his chances of being born would be pretty good. If his mother were over 35, or if she were under 35 and concerned about having a disabled child, she would be offered screening for Down's syndrome, but not usually pressured into such screening. After Adam was born, the county-based habilitation team would be assigned to our family, as well as the normal visits from health and social care professionals that surround any birth. We would be given advice to apply for support under LSS, and possibly financial help under LASS (and would use our right to appeal if the decision was not favourable). If we were not very good at 'pushing' for things for Adam, information about what is available would still have a high chance of reaching us, as would assistance in applying for support. With Adam having Down's syndrome, it would be clear what he, and we, would be entitled to, and therefore a high chance that we would get it. Adam would go to places in the daytime where he would meet other young children (either with or without us being there) and he would be known to our municipality as he came up to the age where education services would be available.

Educational Services – special school within the mainstream?

Given the number of times the all-embracing nature of the welfare state in Sweden has been mentioned already, it will come as no surprise to readers that the education system is overwhelmingly one provided by the state, and is laid out in a rational fashion, with central policies being interpreted and administered at local level by the municipalities. Independent schools do exist in Sweden, for around 6 per cent of compulsory school age students (Government Offices of Sweden 2007), but these are largely organized on the basis of a particular religious or educational philosophy, rather than simply being independent of the mainstream system, and they must follow the approved curriculum and be registered by the government. Compulsory education runs from the ages of 7–16, but educational services are provided from pre-school age (especially for 6-year-olds) up to 20 years of age, with the latter part being called (in English) 'Upper secondary'. This total system applies equally to children with identified intellectual disabilities as to other children, but with additional elements for the former group. Prior to 1994, a completely separate syllabus existed for pupils with intellectual disabilities, and they were taught in schools run at county level. From 1994, a national curriculum for 'compulsory education' has applied to all pupils, with 'special school programmes' being adapted to fit in with the overall curriculum and in 1998 the curriculum was amended to cover pre-school classes and leisure-time centres in schools. All this has resulted in the following options normally being offered to parents of children with intellectual disabilities, as they go through the various age bands.

- *Pre-compulsory education* – in the form of pre-schools, family daycare homes and open pre-schools up to the age of 6, then, for 6-year-olds, a free 'pre-school class' programme, normally at a regular school.
- *Compulsory schooling* – the nine compulsory school years, either in a 'compulsory school', i.e. a regular primary or secondary school, or in a 'training school', depending on assessment and parental choice. Children with intellectual disabilities may also take a tenth year at compulsory school.
- *Childcare for schoolchildren* – provided for children from 6 years until 12 years of age and operated in after-school centres, family daycare homes and open recreational activity centres, mostly integrated with school activities.
- *Upper secondary education* – like all young people after compulsory school, pupils with intellectual disabilities are offered education at the 'upper secondary' level, i.e. between the ages of 17 and 20. Again a separate programme exists for these pupils, but within a national curriculum, and there are a number of nationally designed programmes of a pre-vocational nature that are very similar for all pupils. In addition, like all adults, adults with intellectual disabilities may return to school or college to take basic vocational training programmes.

Looking in more detail at the above system, reflecting on my visits, and comparing Sweden with many other countries, three points immediately stand out. First, the degree of specification of *programmes*, for all pupils, regardless of which *school* they may attend. Second, the high proportion of children attending *free, municipally provided*, education programmes. Third, obviously related to point one, the *lack of competition* between schools or even, to that extent, between pupils, in terms of 'results' (the word 'results' elsewhere tends to mean results of externally set and graded academic assessments). The implications of these points of difference for children with intellectual disabilities are, I believe, significant.

From point one, the choice of *school* for a child with an intellectual disability becomes less significant than the assessment of that child for a particular *curriculum*. The national guidelines state that the assessment should be co-ordinated by a nominated officer of the local authority, involve the parents and family of the child very closely, and assess the following aspects, in terms of needed support

- *education* – whether the child can achieve the curriculum;
- *psychological* – the child's intellectual capacity;
- *medical* – any possible medical reasons for the child's difficulties and their implications for the future;
- *social* – issues outside school.

The results of this assessment determine whether a child is (1) said to need the 'special schooling' programme; and (2) whether this needs to be in a 'practical training school', i.e. a physically separate school for people defined as being more severely intellectually disabled, with a significantly different timetable and subjects which emphasize what is seen to be appropriate for them, namely 'creative activities, communication, motor skills, everyday activities, and conception of reality'.

Most children defined under (1) above, however, will attend a regular secondary school, with varying degrees of integration into the classes attended by children not on the special programme.

From my visit to various parts of the school system, a similar impression to other aspects of Swedish services emerged, which emphasizes the second point of reflection noted above. This is that the existence of a relatively homogeneous, freely available, school system is the result of, and reinforces, *trust* in the decisions made by the 'professionals' regarding whether children go on the 'special schooling' list. This trust may also be partly because of the involvement of parents with professionals from early days of a child's life, noted above, but I would suggest that it also stems from my third point above, that there is less competition between schools. Schools are not generally 'graded' according to externally assessed results, nor do they seem to be the subject of competition between parents, at least not on the sole criteria of academic achievement.

The secondary school I visited described itself as 'popular' with parents of children with intellectual disabilities. The Head of the 'special programme' has the title of 'Assistant Headteacher', and is part of the management team of the school, but has her own staff for the 'special programme' who will have done an extra 2–3 years of training in teaching intellectual disability groups. The school gets more resources per head for these pupils, which also covers a number of personal 'assistants'. The classes are physically part of the larger school, but numbers in each of the nine class groups are somewhat lower. Those I observed for the 'special programme' ranged from five children with Down's syndrome in one group, to about eight or nine children with very mild issues in the 'top' group. Regular classes had about 20–30 children in each. The curriculum followed, as noted above, is a modified version of the national timetable, with 'academic' subjects one would normally expect at a secondary school supplemented by more vocationally oriented subjects. These latter are also taken as part of the regular curriculum and therefore many of the classes are integrated; in fact, the 'vocational' element of the educational system as a whole struck me, as an outsider, as having a much greater credibility than I had come across elsewhere, so that the students on the 'special programme' did not stand out as being the only ones doing such subjects.

Finally, at 'upper secondary level', there is again the system of a 'special programme' within the physical space of the regular system, though this is different for those at 'training schools' – the more severely disabled group. Nearly all 'compulsory school' students stay on at the 'upper secondary' level, and the vocational element for all continues. Again viewing this as an outsider, it appears that access to the post-secondary and university system in Sweden is considerably less of a 'rat race' than in some countries (including the UK), and that schools are not judged on how many of their pupils go on to post-secondary education. The element of competition that can elsewhere 'crowd out' attention to those pupils not 'achieving academically' at the end of their schooling, especially those with intellectual disabilities, is much less in evidence in Sweden. Upper secondary education for students on the 'special programme' route offers vocational training in the form of national, specially designed, or individual programmes, similar to those of regular upper secondary students, though four years in length rather than three. The national programmes for students with intellectual disabilities are also fewer in number and specially oriented to vocational training. As we shall see below, such programmes fit with the pattern of day services that are likely to be offered to young people as they leave the school system. Before considering that, however, a further thought on Adam's World Tour is given.

ADAM'S WORLD TOUR

Going to school in Sweden

If Adam were now coming up to the age of 6 in Sweden, he would almost certainly have been attending pre-school services, in one or other of the various options for such services, preferably a local school. There, we would have been advised to apply for Adam to be assessed for the 'special school' programme. In view of the resources such an assessment would generate, and the fact that his intellectual disability was a 'known' one, then the result of the assessment would be quite predictable. Given the presence of most people with Down's syndrome in the regular 'compulsory school' system, we would probably have also been advised that it would be most likely that, once assessed as needing 'special school' , Adam would be in a regular class for most of the time at primary level (up to 11) though with some activities in a separate group. We would also possibly have been advised, depending on our location, that our local primary school was a 'feeder' school for a secondary school that would be likely to include Adam in one of their 'special programme' classes, and that the friends that he made at the primary school would probably move on with him to the secondary school.

If we were insistent that Adam went to a primary school that had not been recommended, perhaps because it was located nearer to our home, or perhaps his brothers were attending, we would have the right to do so, though if it did not have many, or any, 'special programme' students, we would be under some pressure to place Adam elsewhere. This would, we would be advised, not be a usual occurrence, and certainly we would expect there to be a local secondary school with a significant group of students on the 'special programme' where Adam could go at 11. At such a school, Adam would almost certainly be in a 'special programme' class, perhaps with several other pupils with Down's syndrome, and would have a mixture of the national curriculum and a particular set of individual options, depending on his preferences and abilities. After the age of 17, Adam would be offered a place at an 'upper secondary school' with the possibility of carrying out one of the elements of the 17 national programmes that relate to vocational education. Here, he would possibly work alongside students not on the 'special programme' route, but also be part of classes only containing such students. He would be noted on the municipality's list of potential school leavers as he came up to 20 or 21, and plans would be made for his progression to day services.

Adam would therefore have gone through the school system alongside children with and without intellectual disabilities, though more frequently in the company of those on the 'special programme' route as he got older. The chance of his making friends, whose friendship went beyond and after school, would be significant, though more likely those friends would be other young people with intellectual disabilities.

Adult education

As we saw earlier, all students have the right to begin an upper secondary education in a regular school until the year they turn 20 (or 21 in some cases for people with intellectual disabilities). After that, there are different types of municipally run adult education programmes. Among these are municipal adult education (*Komvux*) and education for adults with intellectual disabilities (*Sarvux*). Though mostly offered in a non-school environment, *Komvux* and *Sarvux* cover both 'basic education', corresponding to compulsory school programmes and programmes for pupils with intellectual disabilities respectively, and 'non-compulsory education', corresponding to regular upper secondary and upper secondary courses for students with intellectual disabilities. The key difference at the adult level is that courses are individually selected, and it is important to repeat the impression of the significant credibility of pre-vocational courses in Sweden, noted in the reflections on secondary school programmes. Students with intellectual disabilities may find themselves studying in the same place as staff who work in the service system who may need to take the pre-vocational courses in 'health and social care' that are normally required for permanent employment in that system. As far as adults with intellectual disabilities are concerned, however, given that such courses are now readily available at upper secondary school, the impression came over that the adult education versions are more used by older adults. For this group, opportunities when they were at school were not as broad as those offered to their younger counterparts. Most school leavers these days will therefore be more likely to move from school into one of the following two sorts of daytime services.

Daytime services – non-work – therapy rules?

From the very beginning of their dealings with the professional service world, people with severe and complex needs in Sweden would appear to have access to a full range of what might be grouped together under the heading of 'therapeutic' services. This continues, with input still from the county habilitation team, during time at the 'training schools'. Some habilitation teams, such as the one I visited, organize themselves into a 'Children and Youth' section (up to the age of 20) and then an 'Adult' team, though they are all part of the overall habilitation effort.

At the age of 20 or 21 when they leave school, therefore, the general picture for people with such multiple disabilities appears to be that they continue to receive 'therapy' services, at least as far as daytime provision is concerned. They will often go on to the sort of day centre I visited, though the particular building may not be typical. It was, in fact, the 'day' part of an old institution, a huge building with various sensory rooms, therapy pool, water beds, etc. Everyone using this centre is supposed to have an individual programme, and for this group of people there is a high staff ratio, with a number of people working there with an OT qualification after the basic social care course at school. For a total of 15 people attending in the morning and 9 in the afternoon, the building seemed vast, and it is true that similar programmes in other parts of the country have smaller, more recently built sites for these sorts of services (Tideman 2005). Regardless of the building, they normally contain, on the whole, what would be regarded in some countries as a vast amount of equipment for so few people, but this does seem to mean individual programmes can be carried out. The local co-ordinator said it was 'not the best but not the worst' compared to other centres elsewhere.

Some people attend both these sort of therapeutic centres and also the self-contained 'workshops' which others with less severe needs attend, and some programmes look to serve all groups of people with an aim towards what is called 'work'. This raises the somewhat artificial nature of my division in Table 2.1 above, between 'work-related' and 'non- work-related' daytime services, which will return in all of the countries of this book, and this is compounded by the entitlement under LSS. The *Socialstyrelsen* summary of the relevant section is

10. *Daily activities* – People of working age who have no gainful employment and are not on a course, are entitled to daily activities if they are part of groups 1 and 2 under the LSS.

(Socialstyrelsen 2006: 1)

A look back at the three groupings will show that Group 3 under LSS would be called 'more able' but the sorts of services provided for this group, and many in Group 2, though not of the 'therapy' kind, could not necessarily be called 'gainful employment', though they have significant 'work' elements. This confusion may be clarified as we move on to look at what I have called 'work-related services'.

Daytime services – work – is it what you do or the fact you get paid?

In their published material (e.g. Mica 2005; SDV 2005), day services in Sweden do not make the distinction that I have between 'work' and 'non-work'. The assessment of the municipal co-ordinator, made prior to school leaving, recommends a place in one of a number of 'day centres'. In most places this day centre placement is meant to be geographical, i.e. near the person's residence, but the practice seems to be, as we have seen above, that the less able are recommended for places at those centres that have the equipment and the specialists. The assessments do not appear to follow a uniform process, but all, following LSS, are supposed to include an individual plan if this is requested. Of course, this may well have been done at a much earlier age, and the daytime activities will only be an update.

As elsewhere, however, the reality is one of available places and forms of day centre, and thus the process also has an element of fitting people to the range of services that exist. Day centres set their activities according to the overall planning process for the municipality as a whole, then the plan of the intellectual disability specialism, then the plan of the centre, all of which are public documents. In practice, this seems to result in a fairly uniform programme of 'contract work', and some developmental activities, within the segregated centres, most of which take 40–50 people with high staff ratio. People seem to stay there – the buildings are not purpose-built, and tend to be rented office or workspaces in the towns and cities. In rural areas, such centres can be based on farms, and involve people in the sort of agricultural and gardening activities that fit the conditions.

A growing trend, (e.g. Mica 2005; SDV 2005) seems to be for people to be placed in what are officially called 'Community-related daily activities' though this is interpreted in different ways in different authorities. Some include all day centres as part of the process, and consider the industrial type work carried out in 'sheltered' conditions as part of the brief. Others use the day centres as a base, and send out 'work groups' to undertake tasks in commercial concerns. Yet others extend this practice to place individuals in regular commercial concerns, though not on the same terms as regular employees. It is possible for people with intellectual disabilities to enter what could be called 'open employment', most often through the employment finding service that places people with other disabilities, but this has a dramatic effect on the level of benefits and other assistance that exist under the Swedish system. One person I spoke to described the situation as people almost 'defining themselves out' of the service world by taking up open employment.

Such a range of activities brings us back to the deeper and more nuanced reflections on what is 'real work'. To aid our reflections, however, it may be worth describing two of the schemes of 'work-type' activity that I observed on my visit. In Jonkoping, I was taken to a 'café' in the town hall run by the 'SDV' part of the municipal day services. This service, as well as having its own 'sheltered workshop' in the form of an independent company called 'Samhall' that combines assembly-based contract work with what is called 'training', sends out people, mostly in groups and with supervisors from the day services staff, into what they describe, in the English translation of their brochure as 'integration of individuals or groups on regular places of work where special, but meaningful, activities are created' (SDV 2005). The phrase 'special but meaningful' became clearer as I visited the café, and then later in my trip to the town of Ostersund. In effect, it means people doing work in regular places of employment that does not replace existing workers, but creates something useful for the place in which it occurs. Thus the café in the town hall would not have been there but for the programme, but is both a useful and valued addition to the place where both civil servants and politicians (especially the city 'cabinet') work. So, like others in this part of the day services, people were doing real work in terms of the jobs that they carried out, but were not paid a wage for doing so. A small allowance, referred to as 'pay' is given to people in addition to their pension, but all people at day centres get this. I was told that there was not much turnover in work teams, or in movement to paid work, though the plans are, theoretically, reviewed annually. As they get older, people may go back to the day centre, or to a special 'day club'.

A similar system, but serving all people as far as day activities were concerned, was 'Mica' in Ostersund. This agency of the municipality in the north of Sweden took the view, according to their publicity materials, that 'Everyone has the right to work'. Their name, in fact, is the acronym of the Swedish phrase translated as 'Man in the centre – work'. Their focus led to the evolution of what they describe as the '3-step process'. Step 1, carried out at their own centres, is essentially an assessment of people and then a 'try-out' of skills for different work possibilities. Step 2 is real work with supervision, either as part of a group or individually, in the sort of places attended by those from the Jonkoping SDV, with monitoring of progress and more trying out of different tasks. Step 3 is where the person is more closely integrated into a company, and more able to work on their own, but it can still be as part of a group at the same stage. A list of the sort of places used by Mica (2005) shows a greater number than Jonkoping, reflecting perhaps the greater work focus of the former, though it may be more an issue of administration and organization than an issue of possibilities to reach 'real' employment, since the basic issues of 'sheltered work' remain. These 'special but meaningful' work activities appear to be increasing within day services in Sweden. It was reported to be the main area of growth in the Jonkoping day service system, and Mica were in great demand from elsewhere in Sweden to present information on their system. Standing back from the highly positive imagery of people doing real, valued work, in real valued workplaces, the question, as far as benefits to people with intellectual disabilities are concerned, is how significant is the *paid* aspect of that work, including the imagery associated with having equal status with one's fellow workers. This is another question that will come up again in future chapters, and clearly has connections to the relative value given by the different societies to 'work', in the sense of the *activities and location* of 'real work in real places' or 'work', in the sense of *'a fair day's pay for a fair day's work'*. In Sweden, it is the observation of this outsider that the 'Protestant work ethic' is alive and well, and therefore the former sense of the value of work as an end in itself is seen by Swedish society as important. Value is thus given to people 'doing work', with the payment issue secondary, especially when it is pragmatically pointed out that people, despite not being paid the 'going rate' are still financially equal, if not better off, than those few people with intellectual disabilities who have obtained paid jobs in the open employment market.

Residential services – are there still 'institutions of the mind?'

The above phrase comes from Ericsson (2000), cited in the history section. That history, as in all the countries, is dominated by the movements against, and total or partial closure of, large segregated institutions, and we have seen how Sweden strongly asserts (and has legislated for) their closure to be complete. My observations and reading would tend to bear out the success of this policy, certainly in the sense of no institutions. What, however, has replaced them in terms of residential services? In the view of most writers on the Swedish scene, e.g. Tideman (2005), the term 'group home' appears to be the most frequently used, and this is unfortunate, as the term means different things in different countries. LSS uses the following phrase in point 9 of its list of rights, allowing for a range of options.

> 9   *Residential arrangements with special service for adults, or other specially-adapted residential arrangements* – These can be various arrangements but the most common types are group homes and service homes. The individual may also be entitled to specially-adapted housing to which they are referred by the municipality.

Of course, LSS supplements other entitlements of all citizens in Sweden. The Social Services Act of 2002, as well as tightening up on the ability to appeal against decisions about assistance and applying new regulations regarding fees for disabled care, re-emphasized the duty of municipal Social Services to inform, and make available to 'functionally disabled individuals' a range of services that could be called 'residential'. Focusing specifically for a moment on those services directly involved in the physical settings where people live, a Socialstyrelsen advice document on the 2002 Social Services Act gives a clear description of what is normally offered, and it is, in fact very straightforward. From a larger list, these three points tell the story

- *specially adapted apartments* with support facilities, such as home help services or personal assistance;
- *group accommodation or an apartment in a special housing complex*, for individuals who want and need to have staff available 24 hours a day;
- *home help services* or home-based assistance in the form of service, practical assistance or personal care.

(Socialstyrelsen 2002: 23)

The person with Down's syndrome whose story started this chapter was an example of the third of these systems, in that her flat was not provided directly by the municipality, but she did have assistance for getting up and for other aspects of home life, though without live-in staff. In my discussions with parents in Jonkoping, I was told of two young women, in their mid-twenties, who were moving into an apartment together, having been friends since schooldays. The process involved an application, from the young women but with help from parents, who also made out a case for the level of support their daughters required. They had been offered a lower level than they had requested, but one which they felt able to accept, and the young women and their parents had been looking for apartments. They had no physical disabilities requiring adaptations, so the only issue was the 'standard price' that the municipality set for the sort of apartment they wanted. This would cover apartments in certain areas, but not where these particular people (or their parents) wanted them to be. So it was possible to make up the difference in the rental to get what they wanted, and the young women were due to move in soon.

Given, therefore, that the range of housing options is pretty much limited, in a physical sense, to 'ordinary' apartments or houses, then it is only the choice between 'group accommodation' and individual apartments that seems to be the issue. Visiting one of the former types in Jonkoping, even this was physically not very different from the individual apartment in the university block in which I was staying. From the outside, the 'group accommodation' residence did not stand out from the other apartments in the complex, and even inside the only difference was a central lounge area that led off to the four individual apartments of the residents. As for the 'group' nature of the residence, and how it was made up, what emerged was the familiar story of attempts to match 'compatible' people, but with the limitations of a finite number of spaces, and the economic demands of minimum numbers of 'empty beds'. As far as the aims of the service were concerned, therefore, the key fact of the group apartment, as for the individual apartments or the assistance in one's own home, was that it was physically integrated with 'normal' housing, and that residents had their individual space.

'Non-direct' services – the source of real integration?

In the last four rows of Table 2.1 are listed an uneasy collection of items which, while they could be said to be 'services' in the sense that they are supports to people to pursue ordinary lives, are not always named as such, or listed in catalogues or budget headings of the formal service system. On the other hand, their quantity and quality seemed to me to be important in all the countries visited, both in their own right, but also in the way in which they put pressure on, and complement, the basic services of education, daytime activity for adults, and residential provision.

The first, *financial assistance*, sometimes determines whether individuals can, in fact, pursue independent lives with an element of choice and control, or whether they are effectively tied to particular services by powerful economic pressures. Thus we have seen the effect of the pension levels and subsidies to housing on the incentive to move into full-time paid employment, but also on the ability of those people with substantial needs to still be able to live in ordinary accommodation. There is other financial assistance in the form of home adjustment grants for modifications to physical settings, and assistance with transport for both parents and people themselves, though the rules vary according to the municipality. Overall, however, the combination of services, mostly paid for through municipal funds, financial assistance via the pension system and LASS to pay for direct personal assistance, provides, in my view, a comprehensive set of supports for most people with intellectual disabilities.

Support for *leisure*, as we have seen, is also indirectly specified through LSS, especially the support elements of items 1–4 listed above, though the long history of the meeting places or 'clubs' provided by FUB still gives them a key role in the leisure time of many people. Given concerns over safety, and the all-pervasive nature of services, events in people's lives do not occur 'naturally' or spontaneously as often as their non-disabled peers. The logistics and support needed by people even to simply 'hang out', or to do something on the spur of the moment or out of the ordinary routine tends to mean that such things happen less often, as a number of studies have shown (Ringsby-Jansson 2002; Tideman 2005). As we shall see later, however, this appears to be a universal issue for community-based services for people with intellectual disabilities, and the sheer fact of an entitlement to assistance with leisure would be looked on with envy by parents elsewhere.

Less prominent, though with a longer history than many places, are services that could be called *advocacy*. The history, of course, relates to the combination of parents' groups that formed FUB, and early attempts at what could be called 'self-advocacy' by people such as Nirje. This will prove a much bigger issue in some other countries, where the dealings between parents and the service system is less trusting than in Sweden, and also where the notion of the rights of individual people with intellectual disabilities to have the key say in decisions affecting their lives has greater prominence than I observed in that country. FUB certainly organizes conferences and other ways in which people with intellectual disabilities can meet and discuss issues more broadly, and, as we have seen, the views of individual adults are supposed to be prominent in things like where they want to work and/or live. The overall impression, however, is still that parents have significant power, even when their offspring are adults, and broader policies, while consultation with parents, and people themselves seems good, are still strongly the province of the 'professionals' (FUB 1999).

Finally, we come to that most nebulous and controversial of topics, even in the way I have named it, that of *parental services*. It should be clear by now that the Swedish welfare state, like all the countries discussed in this book, relies on parents playing an active role in matters that affect their offspring when they are children. This is a truism of all industrialized countries with anything resembling a welfare system, but the extra effort and involvement of parents of children with intellectual disabilities, and then a continuation of that responsibility into their adulthood, are much more varied. In Sweden, the issue seems, as noted a number of times now, to relate to the long-standing welfare state, and its maintenance of trust between citizens and government. If services are seen as an entitlement of citizenship, rather than as the compensation for some 'deficit' in the person, then the devaluation of people with intellectual disabilities, while still a universal tendency in modern societies, seems to me to be lessened. The role of parents in ensuring those entitlements of citizenship, while again not a trivial matter, is, I would argue, considerably eased by the continuing existence of the fully fledged welfare state in Sweden. The possible downside of that easing of total responsibility is, I would suggest, an acceptance, at least in large part, of the power of the state to determine what are 'quality services'. Though it appears that consultation is good, especially from a parent's perspective, what is provided is largely determined by the prescription of LSS, itself largely written by the professional service system, and by the local implementation of that by the municipalities.

Despite this possible criticism, we shall see in later chapters how parents in other countries would look with envy at what is available to their counterparts in Sweden, and see, in our final thoughts on Adam's life as an adult in Sweden, many things for which they can only wish, pray and/or fight.

ADAM'S WORLD TOUR

An adult citizen of Sweden

Given Adam's likely experiences were he at school in Sweden, he would be on the list of the municipality for plans to be made, when he was around the age of 18/19, for what would happen after school. Assuming he, or we as his parents, called for a formal review of the plan that had come through the school system with him, we would be part of this process; with Adam, the assessor from the municipality, and others that they or we requested. In most places, Adam would be recommended, either to a day centre, from where he would go out on 'work experience' or with that part of the day service system that involved people in the world of work. Depending on the process, and Adam's wishes and skills, this could lead to a fairly settled place in the working world, though the notion of Adam working entirely in the open market would be much more rarely discussed, despite remaining a possibility. If Adam wanted to set up in an apartment of his own, or share with one or two friends, the municipality would have to consider (this could have been part of the plan above) the level of support he might need. We as parents would be consulted, and possibly look to contribute towards costs if we (or Adam) wanted a property with a higher cost than that suggested by the municipality. If we took very little interest as parents, or even did not think he should leave home, Adam might well still be offered the chance to set up in an apartment under the LSS law. In either case he would then have a social life that could be helped by free or cheap transport, a 'support person', 'companion', 'personal contact' and/or one of the social clubs run by FUB, where his friends from school would likely be attending. If he met someone he wanted a more intimate relationship with, then support in this would probably be given, though we as parents might have a say in what happened. If he had more severe disabilities, then he would be more likely to attend a more therapeutic day service, and probably move to a 'group home', where he would have his own part of an apartment or house shared with two or three other people.

3　Norway

Big brother's shadow or going the extra mile?

Tweedledum and Tweedledee
Agreed to have a battle;
For Tweedledum said Tweedledee
Had spoiled his nice new rattle.

Just then flew down a monstrous crow,
As black as a tar-barrel;
Which frightened both the heroes so,
They quite forgot their quarrel.

(Lewis Carroll)

INSTANT IMPACTS

Norway – mine host

In my last evening in Norway, I took my host out for a meal. Partly randomly, and partly on the suggestion of another 'SRV person' in the city, we went to what was described as 'trendy' restaurant, whose ambience I would call 'designer basic', i.e. carefully placed bare wood tables and chairs in the two small rooms of the working-class cottage from which it had been converted. Fortunately early, we could observe of the steady stream of people who arrived for a meal, mostly young students, but also others who in Paris would have been described (by the English) as 'bohemian' types. A waitress came to take our order, a young lady in her thirties, who also happened to have Down's syndrome. Writing the order down, she laid our places, and later delivered the food. As with all my visits, I had talked to different people, read many documents, and visited a number of services. I had also, over many years, seen people with learning disabilities in open employment, so why would this stick in my mind as an 'Instant Impact'. I think it was mainly because, despite the many advances in services in Norway, they, like Sweden, had not totally cracked the open employment riddle. I had seen, in both countries, people doing 'regular work'. But, largely because of the way the benefit system operates and the agreement with the unions (a powerful force in Scandinavia though on a more co-operative basis than in many other countries) on the sort of jobs available to disabled people, very few people get paid a regular wage. This young lady was the exception, as was the owner of the restaurant. The story I was told of him was that he had been a postgraduate student in the disability area, and had produced a dissertation demonstrating, from an economic perspective backed up with quantitative data, that it was possible to employ disabled people on full wages, and still run a viable business. Though his thesis was, I gather, received well academically, it did not have an effect on the service system, so he decided to do something himself. Hence the restaurant and mine host with Down's syndrome.

Introduction – an independent welfare state

Travelling by train from Jonkoping to Oslo, my first brief port of call in Norway, for a weekend break before the longer ride up through the mountains to Trondheim, the experience of crossing from one country to another was minimal. Architecture and landscape did not seem to vary much, until the large urban sprawl of Oslo came like canyons of apartments to surround the train. As Norway was the only country of the six I was visiting that was completely new to me, I took the normal tourist route over the weekend, of cathedrals, palaces and museums; with my personal preference for cities to be on waterways fully satisfied by the harbour at Oslo's foot. What this harbour area also contained, however, was the old city fortifications and 'war-resistance museum'. That well-laid out (and, mercifully, lingually accessible) building contained clues to what, on reflection, seems to me to be a key issue with regard to the two Scandinavian countries and the small but significant differences between them (hinted at in the opening quotation). This concerns the fact that, in living memory, invasion, including an element of felt betrayal by one group of citizens against another, had, of the two countries, only been experienced by Norway.

What have these reminiscences to do with services? It is my speculation, supported by writers who had been through the Second World War (Derry 1973) that the experience of invasion, and more importantly imprisonment in one's own country, created a major set of cultural beliefs, in those who survived it, regarding two things: first, the independence of the country and its sense of nationhood. This seemed, in Norway, to have been immensely strengthened by coming through the occupation, including a continued highly popular role for the monarchy, as having 'suffered with the people'.

Second, a belief in social justice, easy to ridicule as hollow rhetoric in many countries who speak of the concept while maintaining gross inequalities. In Norway, acceptance of the pre-war welfare state and relatively flat hierarchy of society that we noted in Chapter 1, seems to have been reinforced by the sense of *injustice* generated by invasion. In addition, however, invasion seems to have generated a reaction against *incarceration*, relevant to the growing awareness of the Scandinavian leaders in intellectual disability of the undesirability of institutions.

I was to find a great many similarities with Sweden as regards the administration of services, the sort of facilities in which they were provided, the debates about paternalism of the state, and the historical development of provision. All of this will be outlined below, but it remains an impression that the similarities were tempered somehow by a subtle difference in the sense of independence. This is perhaps also reflected by Norway still remaining, by referendum of its citizens, outside the European Union and, of course, in its separation, as a nation, from the enforced union with Sweden being only just over a hundred years old.

Historical development of services – from segregation to normalization, Social Role Valorization, and beyond

Early developments

By strange coincidence, my visit to Trondheim coincided with that of the Archbishop of Canterbury, Dr Rowan Williams. He was visiting Trondheim, the old capital with its cathedral dating back to 1070, to celebrate the ninth anniversary of the signing of an agreement between the Church of Norway, which, like most Scandinavian churches, is essentially from the Lutheran Protestant tradition, and the Church of England. The role of the Church is, I believe, a key issue in determining the sort of attitudes that have continued to affect the historical development of services to people with intellectual disabilities. Until recently, the ministry involved with education, the area where, like many European countries, those few services that did exist before the twentieth century were grounded, was called the Ministry for Education, Research and Church Affairs.

In terms of what might be called 'state' services, then, these did not really come into being until the turn of the twentieth century. By this time, as we saw in Chapter 1, Norway as a nation was on a par socially with most of Europe, with both democratic governance and the monarchy being established in the Constitution of 1814, full parliamentarianism introduced in 1884, and full nationhood arriving with the separation of the union with Sweden in 1905. As the independent nation looked to establish its identity, issues to do with 'racial purity' and resistance to 'foreign' mixing became entangled, as elsewhere, with the debates on intellectual disability and mental illness under the emerging eugenics furore.

In predominantly rural economies, such as Sweden and Norway, the impact of the Industrial Revolution could be said to have come rather later than some countries, though by the late nineteenth century the development of universal education was, also as elsewhere, beginning to identify more people as of limited intellectual development. This then fed into Norway's particular contribution to the eugenics debate.

Eugenics – science versus populism in Norway

The arguments and 'scientific' rationale for eugenics as a policy have already been outlined in Chapter 2, as has the existence of the small but influential groups who promoted the ideas. The contribution of Norway to this debate was largely of the same kind, particularly in terms of the more populist versions of the 'eugenic danger'. Two issues, however, give some nuanced difference to the Norwegian experience of this important period in the development of attitudes to, and services for, people with intellectual disabilities. First, the fact that there was some dispute, again within the relatively small academic and policy-making circles that had such a powerful influence on European and English-speaking societies, between what might be seen as an 'academic-scientific' group and 'populist-scientific' individuals. This then had an effect on the second aspect of eugenic policy peculiar to Norway, which was noted at the beginning of this chapter, namely the impact of the invasion of Norway, at the 'invitation' of the government of Vidkunn Quisling.

Space does not permit a full account of the personalities involved in the first issue, which can be found, with an interesting and wide-ranging discussion on broader issues of the eugenics movement in Norway, in Roll-Hansen (1996), but two individuals can be used to represent the two 'camps'. Jon Alfred Hansen Mjøen, a pharmacist, had studied abroad, where his interest in 'race hygiene' was stimulated and developed in Germany. In 1901, he was elected a member of the Norwegian Academy of Science and in 1906 founded a private research institute for eugenics, Vinderen Biological Laboratory. Though, according to Roll-Hansen (1996: 155), this 'never developed into a scientific institution of any importance', Mjøen became influential as a propagandist for eugenics, first when he spoke before the Medical Society in Oslo on 'Race Biology and Hygiene of Reproduction', presenting an early version of what later came to be known as 'The Norwegian Programme for Race Hygiene'. In 1914, Mjøen published a popular book on the subject, which was criticized by a number of medical academics, including a young medical doctor, Otto Lous Mohr. Mohr had received his medical degree in 1912 and studied cytology abroad during the year 1913–14. He criticized Mjøen for being a *dilettante* in medicine and biology, and for obscuring important issues and misleading the public by spreading unrealistic hopes about the effectiveness of the proposed eugenic measures.

This therefore represents the essence of what debate there was in Norway; not between those opposed to eugenics and those in favour of it, but merely between those who saw themselves as bounded by empiricism, in what they were suggesting as policy, and those who extrapolated from tentative findings to reach powerful and far-reaching policy implications. Mohr was not against eugenics in general and he did not react to what would now be seen as the racist tendencies in Mjøen's book, merely recommending an alternative book by a leading psychiatrist, Ragnar Vogt (Vogt 1914) as being a more scientifically reliable alternative to Mjøen.

Mjøen's supporters, who were mostly non-medical people, though well placed in society, adopted the growing popular trend of 'enlightenment through science', and objected to what they saw as the smugness and arrogance of the 'scientific' critics. This would all have been a somewhat esoteric debate had not similar comments on eugenics from around the world by non-scientists, but powerful people, which we noted in Chapter 2, made the subject important in policy and legal terms. In particular, though there were disagreements about some of the groups classed as 'inferior', obviously coming to a head with the growing activities in Germany, all sides of the argument agreed that people with intellectual disabilities were part of the 'problem' group. This also, in the early stages of discussion up to and after the First World War, tended to result in two key points of action. First, segregation of people with intellectual disabilities in institutions, and, second, the various policies on sterilization in the different countries. On the former, as in many countries, existing institutions in Norway were expanded and new ones built, though given the rural nature and relatively small population of the country as a whole, the size of these facilities was not as great as some of the other countries, and also included what is loosely translated as 'work-farms' where the segregated nature did not prevent the 'more able' from contributing economically, an important issue in the view of a society that was, and is, seen as the embodiment of the 'Protestant work ethic' (Weber 2005).

Developments on the legalization of sterilization, however, though widely discussed in eugenics circles in North America and Europe, did not come to fruition in as many countries as they might have done. In Norway, ironically, proposals for a law on sterilization from the 'scientific' side of the earlier debate were partly based on the grounds that if it were carried out, then people could be returned from the institutions to the community. Government bodies then debated and heard submissions, most notably from a self-appointed group set up by Mjøen, grandly entitled the Norwegian Consultative Eugenics Committee. Their key proposals were that, in order to prevent 'psychically abnormal' persons from procreating at the current rate, compulsory segregation and voluntary sterilization should be introduced. As a means of segregation, continuation of the institutions and rural work camps were proposed, and, as noted earlier, persons who were not thought to be 'dangerous to society' in other ways could regain freedom by undergoing voluntary sterilization.

Eventually sterilization, either on social grounds, because the prospective parent was 'unfit' to take care of the child, or on genetic grounds, because there was a likelihood that a hereditary disease would be passed on to the child, became law in 1934. One minor passage in the law afforded a small concession to individual rights of people with an intellectual disability. This specified that a 'mentally disabled' person could not be sterilized without their consent if they had reached or could be expected to reach the 'mental level' of a 9-year-old.

The proposer of the law as it passed through Parliament provides a link to the next particularly Norwegian nuance. Erling Bjørnson was a representative from the Farmers Party (*Bondepartiet*), a strong nationalist, and the son of a Norwegian national poet, Bjørnstjerne Bjørnson. He became a member of the Norwegian Nazi Party after the German Occupation in 1940. Being a farmer himself, Bjørnson compared the management of a country's population to the management of livestock on a farm. He declared a personal preference for a stronger law in the direction of compulsory sterilization, similar to the one been passed in Germany in 1933, and expressed thanks to those who had prepared the Norwegian people so that 'the law today is sure to pass', especially the Norwegian Consultative Committee for Eugenics and 'its untiring leader Dr. Alfred Mjøen, who through the passing of this law will receive the recognition in our country that he has long ago gained abroad' (Roll-Hansen 1996: 175). Significantly Bjørnson did not mention any of the medical or biological experts.

So the law came into effect, with figures for the early years dominated by sterilizations of people with intellectual disabilities. The agricultural connection, and the significant, though far from overwhelming, support for the Norwegian Nazi Party that led to the Quisling government and invasion by Germany, was reflected in the change in the law which the Nazi regime brought about. In 1942, a new law was passed 'for the protection of the race' (*'Lov til vern om folkeætten'*), following a commission headed by the newly appointed Nazi director of the health service, H. Thoralf Ostrem. Members included Klaus Hansen, Professor of Medicine at the University of Oslo, who had been a member of Mjøen's Eugenics Committee, and Gunnar Hiorth, Associate Professor of Genetics at the Agricultural College of Norway. The new law was dominated by the idea that biological inheritance was far more important than environmental factors, extended the range of conditions for sterilization, and allowed for coercion, including physical force. In general terms, it weakened the existing, if slender, protection of individual rights. More subtle, however, was a key change related to an underlying philosophy of the subjection of the individual to the interests of the state, ironically a perspective that many have argued was at the heart of the Scandinavian welfare state project.

The founders of that project, in the 1930s, had maintained the perspective of both scientific rationality and provision for individual rights, but their more vociferous and populist colleagues now used the power of that welfare state to implement their policies, which were much more in tune with their Nazi occupiers. Roll-Hansen (1996: 180) quotes figures showing a near trebling of the number of sterilizations under the Nazi law from the years before occupation. Despite this large rise, it does not appear that there was any significant reaction to the more extreme position taken by the Nazi regime, and in many ways the subtleties of causation and definition could hardly be expected to be of primary concern to an occupied country, where the focus on a growing resistance to both the German occupiers and the collaborating government was likely to have been the paramount priority. The law continued in place after the war, with the prevailing view regarding the need for sterilization of those with intellectual disabilities maintaining its place, despite the emerging excesses of the Nazi regime in Germany gradually being revealed. Claims such as those by Evang (1955) that 'most authors assume that 40–60 per cent of existing feeblemindedness is caused by biological heredity' matched similar views in other countries, such as those put forward in later editions of Tredgold's *Textbook on Mental Deficiency* (Tredgold 1952). The continuation of the sterilization law, amended in 1961 to give slightly more emphasis on individual rights, and still further in 1977, was matched by the continuation of institutionalization and 'farm camp' placement being the state's provision for people with intellectual disabilities into the 1960s and 1970s. The 1977 law emphasized even more strongly the initiative resting with the person to be sterilized or somebody with a close personal relationship to them, but despite this, the situation is still an issue for people with intellectual disabilities (Roll-Hansen 1996). Though the 1977 law was adjusted in 2006, guardians can still apply for sterilization of a disabled person if they are deemed incapable of consent (pers. comm. Johansen 2006).

Normalization and SRV – a difference from Sweden?

We saw, in Chapter 2, Scandinavia taking the lead in the early development of normalization ideas. Though it did not have the 'names', such as Nirje or Bank-Mikkelsen, Norway, as part of the Nordic group of countries with their considerable sharing of ideas and pan-Nordic networks, became fully involved in the development of these ideas (Traustadottir 2006). As we have also seen, some of this occurred at international conferences, especially those of the parents groupings, and though it was formed later than those in Sweden and Denmark, the Norwegian parents association, NFU (the initials of the

Norwegian words *Norsk Forbund for Utviklinshemmede*) founded in 1967, was, according to Kristiansen (1999: 396), a 'major factor in shaping social reform directions and standards'. Initially, as in the other Scandinavian countries, the emphasis placed by normalization on people with intellectual disabilities enjoying the same patterns of life, and the same rights within the welfare state, did not lead to a closure of institutions, more to a growing awareness on the limitations those imposed on achieving normalization's goals. Visits by the Scandinavian leaders to the USA added a realization, on observing the far greater size and worse conditions of US institutions, of the potential path that continuation of institutionalization might bring. This in turn, as we have seen, led to the more general movement, among those countries taking normalization seriously, to move away from institutional care. Kristiansen translates and quotes from a Norwegian government report from as early as 1966, in which its objectives include the statement that disabled people should have

> [the] same standard of living, freedom of choice to plan one's life as others ... to the degree that this is possible ... Society must alter conditions so that people with disabilities receive the medical, pedagogical, and social assistance they need to fully develop their capacities. An important principle in this new way of thinking is Normalization. This means that one should not draw unnecessary lines of separation between the disabled and others with regard to medical and social care, schooling, education, occupation, and general welfare.
>
> (Kristiansen 1999: 397–8)

She goes on to note that 'In the history of Norwegian reform, this policy statement has later been referred to "as an important break with segregative care patterns" (St. Meld. 1967: 4).' In legislative terms, however, it was not until 1988 that the law requiring closure of the institutions came into being. Between those two points the nominal acceptance of normalization at government level had led to a number of reports, though fewer changes. Meyer (2004) notes a reduction in special schools in the 1960s and 1970s, and a similar movement towards institutions being largely for adults, rather than children, citing Romøren (1995) to support his assertion that by the late 1970s there were no children under 16 in institutional care. Kristiansen (1999) puts the 1988 law as finally ending segregated education, but agrees with Meyer that the 1980s saw the last of attempts to provide 'better institutions'. Meyer notes that in other countries, provision that was represented in the 1980s as *alternatives* to institutions; 'small and large group homes', and 'clusters of modular houses with 10–20 residents' were still called *institutions* in Norway, and represented provisions prior to 'non-institutional' provision.

As we shall see in later chapters, his point would certainly apply to a number of the countries in this book.

What was going on in Norway, therefore, was a gradual belief, led philosophically by normalization, in the notion that segregated living, however beautiful, could not meet the real needs of people with intellectual disabilities. It is also worth noting that, like Sweden at this time, governance of services, at least via the institutions, was at the level of the county, rather than the more local *kommune* (again normally translated as 'municipality').

A high level group was therefore commissioned, consisting of academics, policy-makers and senior professionals. Such a review (known as NOU, from the Norwegian *Norges offentlig utredning* (public committee report)) tends to carry considerable weight with government, and this one certainly seems to have a strong input from the normalization adherents. Meyer's (2004) translation of its 'standards of quality assessment', 'basic premises' and 'findings' support this view. On quality, the standards were based on

> (1) the ideological tenets of the principle of normalization, (2) the government's commitment to decentralization of services, (3) the goal of the integration of persons with disabilities, and (4) moving toward a broader definition of developmental disabilities as a target group for services.
>
> (Meyer 2004: 97–8)

NOU then defined their premises as follows:

> We assume that the Norwegian people agree that all human beings have the same worth and that this society is a society for all. Norway should give people with developmental disabilities a chance to be reabsorbed in the local community. This goal leads to a recognition that people with developmental disabilities need more public support than other citizens to compensate for the disabilities because people who have fewer human and material resources require better access to greater resources so that social prosperities can be equalized and adapted.
>
> (Meyer 2004: 98 – Author's translation from Norwegian –
> NOU, no. 34, 1985)

This then led to the NOU conclusions:

1   The circumstances of life and standard of living of persons with developmental disabilities in institutions were unacceptable by basic human, social, and cultural standards.

2   There were no rational reasons to send people out of their neighbour-
     hoods to specialized facilities because of developmental disabilities.
3   The special care organization for persons with developmental dis-
     abilities provided poorer medical pedagogical, social and cultural ser-
     vice in the institutions than what was available in people's local
     community.
4   The political accepted goals of normalization, inclusion and decen-
     tralization could only be realized through local (township) responsi-
     bility. Special care organizations whether small (e.g., 8 persons) or
     large (e.g., 150 persons) worked in opposition to the realization of the
     accepted goals for people with developmental disabilities.
5   The township (municipality) responsibility for people with develop-
     mental disability would limit the extent to which people would
     fall between the cracks or find themselves in the "grey areas" of
     responsibility of direct government entities.
6   Continuing to pour money into institution care would yield only
     marginal effects on the living conditions for the people with develop-
     mental disability, but similar investments in services within townships
     could contribute to significantly better lives for people.

(Meyer 2004: 98 – Author's translation from
Norwegian – NOU no. 34, 1985)

Such was the momentum behind this report that legislation was passed
within three years. In summary, it mandated the closure of all institutions,
moved the responsibility for services to the municipality level, specifying
in some detail what those services should be, and set a time period of three
years for the closure programme. As we will review below, there were also
commitments to training, both in general terms and also in normalization,
and, of relevance in this historical review, training not just in normalization,
but in the developed and revised form of those ideas that Wolfensberger,
beginning in 1983 (Wolfensberger 1983, 1984) called Social Role Valorization.
This has been alluded to briefly in Chapter 2, and will figure in other chapters,
but in terms of the development of Norwegian services it represents a significant difference from its Scandinavian neighbour. Another English observer
(Hill 2001), describes a national debate, led by NFU, in the 'late 1980s', and
describes the resultant '11 principles of NFU' as embodying 'social role
valorization'. Comparing his translation of these principles with Nirje's
(1993) statements quoted in Chapter 2 gives a sense of the subtle differences
between a formulation at least influenced by SRV and one based solely on
normalization.

The 11 principles of NFU

1   Right to life; rejection of pre-natal selection.

2 Right to grow up with families or comparable environment with stable adult contact.
3 Right to pre-school, education in ordinary school at all levels, and to adult education.
4 Home of one's own, lifelong suitability.
5 Employment and meaningful activity.
6 Participation in leisure, culture and holidays according to individual interests.
7 Normal way of life, with properly adapted and adequate assistance.
8 Right to company of others, and to family and sexual life.
9 Participation in decisions that affect own life situation, including everyday family decisions.
10 Families with a person with learning disability at home have right to practical and financial support.
11 Right to an organization to protect their rights.

(from Hill 2001: 10)

At the same time, perhaps as a result of the national debate, the Norwegian Ministry of Social and Health Services funded a national training initiative in 1990 which recognized, in Kristiansen's (1999: 400) words, 'that competency in Normalization was relevant for other "groups in society at risk of being socially excluded" and that "Wolf Wolfensberger's work is of special interest in this regard." '. Though published in the full written proceedings in 1999, Kristiansen's account was actually delivered in May 1994, at the first International SRV conference in Ottawa. By then, Kristiansen notes that nearly 1,000 people had attended 3-day SRV workshops over the previous two years, with a significant number going on to more intensive teaching on workshops based on the evaluation instrument PASS (Wolfensberger and Glenn 1975) and other events with origins in Wolfensberger's Training Institute. There were also a number of publications on SRV in Norwegian, not least by Kristiansen herself (Kristiansen 1993), and the 1990s training and NFU principles are also relevant to the origins of what is now the Nordic Network on Disability Research (NNDR), in that Kristiansen, as one of the significant leaders in the worldwide SRV network, was a member from the early days, and other NNDR activists had attended SRV and PASS training. This appears to be unique when compared with other academic disability networks, especially in the UK, where there appears to have been a dominance of disabled academics and their development of the 'social model' of disability (Barnes et al. 1999; Traustadottir 2006).

Kristiansen's words on the Norwegian experience of this particular focus for training and policy will, we hope, be addressed for all the countries we are looking at, but here they provide the foreword to our more detailed examination of the impression gained of her country's services 11 years after her Ottawa presentation.

Norway remains the only Scandinavian country to have instituted formalized training in Normalization/SRV, including events via the international network, Historians and researchers can assist us in answering the question "So what?"

(Kristiansen 1999: 401)

Services in Norway – an impression

Overview

As we saw in the history above, many Norwegian services are based on national legislation implemented through the municipalities. The size of Norway's population and its geographical distribution mean that such municipalities can range in size from small villages to large cities, with Oslo a significantly special case. The responsibilities, however, in terms of services for people with intellectual disabilities, are the same for municipalities large and small. Table 3.1 below uses our common framework to provide an overview of those services.

Table 3.1 Schematic overview of 'services' that affect the lives of people with intellectual disabilities in Norway

'Service'	Formal organizational place	Specialist or generic?	Main source(s) of funding
Pre-natal services	County health services – Clinics and Habilitation teams	Generic and specialist	Taxation, raised by counties and 'equalized' by central government
Post-natal and early childhood services	County health services – Habilitation teams Municipal early childhood services Norwegian Support System for Special Education	Generic, but with input dependent on individual children	Taxation, raised by counties and municipalities and 'equalized' by central government
Non-educational services for children	Municipal services	Specialist	Taxation, raised by municipalities and 'equalized' by central government – also National Social Insurance payments for personal assistance

Education services – children and young adults	Municipal services County for High Schools (16+) Norwegian Support System for Special Education	Generic and specialist	Taxation, raised by municipalities and 'equalized' by central government
Education services – adults	Municipal services Norwegian Support System for Special Education	Generic and specialist	Taxation, raised by municipalities and 'equalized' by central government
Residential services – adults	Municipal services	Generic and specialist	Taxation, raised by municipalities and 'equalized' by central government
Daytime services – non-work	Municipal services	Largely specialist	Taxation, raised by municipalities and 'equalized' by central government
Daytime services – work	Municipal services	Largely specialist	Taxation, raised by municipalities and 'equalized' by central government
Leisure assistance	Municipal services NFU	Largely specialist	Taxation, raised by municipalities and 'equalized' by central government
Advocacy services	Municipal services NFU	Specialist	Taxation, raised by municipalities and 'equalized' by central government
Financial Assistance	Social Insurance Board	Specialist within generic service	Taxation, distributed to Social Insurance Board by central government
Parental 'support services'	Acting as all parents – not a job in an organization, but can be active in NFU	Specialist, in that all children are different	Own finances, plus some grants via municipalities or Social Insurance Board

Pre-natal services – also bucking the Western trend?

As in Sweden, the reality of Norway's position on pre-natal screening and abortion appeared to defy the 'scientific, rational' image that might have been indicated by its earlier laws on sterilization, in that its services seemed to veer more towards the desirability of the birth of disabled children than is the case in the other five countries. Until 1964, abortions were only permitted in Norway for medical reasons, but then broader criteria came into effect, though abortion could still not be legally performed on socio-economic grounds alone. Such issues could, however, be taken into consideration by a board of approval, with further legislation in 1975 allowing abortions specifically on socio-economic grounds, and an automatic right of appeal against a refusal. The current abortion law has stood since 1978 and this legislation produced further liberalization. If a pregnancy places a woman in 'serious difficulties', she may obtain an abortion on request during the first 12 weeks of pregnancy. The abortion application must be submitted by the woman herself, though if she is defined as having an intellectual disability or a severe mental illness, submission may be by a guardian. If the woman is under 16 or has an intellectual disability, the opinion of a parent or guardian concerning the abortion is also considered. After 12 weeks, a legal abortion must be performed in a hospital and requires the authorization of a committee composed of two physicians, who look at whether

- the pregnancy, childbirth or childcare may result in 'unreasonable strain' on the physical or mental health of the woman or place her in 'difficult circumstances';
- there is a major risk that the child may suffer from a serious disease, which includes some conditions such as Down's syndrome;
- the pregnancy resulted from a criminal act;
- the woman is defined as having a severe mental illness or intellectual disability.

Abortions may not be performed after 18 weeks of pregnancy unless there are particularly important grounds, and if there is reason to assume that the foetus is viable, authorization cannot be granted.

It could therefore be argued that pregnant women with intellectual disabilities do not get much of a say in whether they can carry the pregnancy to term, since, as we have seen, parents or guardians are given an opportunity to express a view with regard to the abortion, and in fact it is usual for applications to be submitted by them. On the other hand, *screening* for potential disability is, like Sweden, usually only given to older women or those with a history of disability in the family. The process is outlined by Irgens (2004), with similar categories of pregnant women being offered tests in the following three instances: screening for Down's syndrome, indications for pre-natal cytogenetic diagnosis, and screening for structural anomalies by ultrasound. In a 2000 survey however, Jakobsen et al. found that 54 per cent of physicians surveyed had *no* patients who had taken predictive tests, only 50 per cent of the same physicians would advise on taking a test if one of the known parents had an inheritance risk, and only 22 per cent were in favour of abortion if a genetic abnormality was detected. This supports the anecdotal evidence of attitudes from a person I met, herself involved in the local health service, but not in this sector. On becoming pregnant in her forties, she was told by her doctor regarding possible screening that 'you won't want to bother with all that, will you?' Like Sweden, this attitude may well be affected by the perceived quality and availability of disability services, and partly by a general attitude towards abortion that is permissive in early pregnancy, but somewhat firmer past the 12 week stage.

Early childhood services – habilitation and early intervention

Similarities with Sweden continue after the birth of a child with an intellectual disability. If the condition is obvious or has been identified pre-birth, then 'habilitation', the health professionals at regional or 'county' level, step in – they work on health issues, but also inform parents regarding the future. The municipality is normally informed within three months of birth, and the full network of professionals, plus parents, appears to be set in motion. The local authority workers co-ordinate what happens with the child at home, though, as in Sweden, they use the 'habilitation' experts for specific health issues. A plan for the child is then built up regarding assistance in the home, education (with workers advising parents on home development, etc.) and then the offer of place in a kindergarten. All children with disabilities are entitled to a kindergarten place, with 'education' via nursery nurses, headed by someone who has taken a 'special needs' option in their training. Specific issues are still addressed by reference to the generic 'habilitation team' who will advise onsite staff, but increasing use is made of regionally based specialists gathered under one administrative body, the *Norwegian Support System for Special Education*. Because they have to deal with a range of educational provision and a range of degrees of rurality, the national system consists of a number of 'units', some operating regionally, some nationally (Odin 2007) but under a single joint board. The units carry out a variety of tasks and are affiliated in different ways to the national support system. Their input, and the national policies for the pre-school child with intellectual disabilities and their parents, seem to provide the kind of support that we have noted in Swedish pre-school services This, together with the practically universal system of state-provided education in Norway, has meant that the planning of educational services, and the degree of national uniformity of provision, seem to place the two Scandinavian countries in a similar position regarding the inclusion of children into mainstream education. We will consider this in more detail below, but continue our reflections on Adam's World Tour before we do so.

ADAM'S WORLD TOUR

Conceived in Norway – what next?

Like Sweden, if Adam were now conceived in Norway, he would have a good chance of being born. If his mother were 38 or over, or there was a history of disability, she would be offered screening for such things as Down's syndrome, but attitudes by local medical practitioners to such screening seem somewhat mixed. After Adam was born, the county-based 'habilitation' team would be involved with our family, and we would be given advice about support from our local authority, who would be advised of Adam's birth within three months. Their worker would take up our case, with the reality of the budgets to which they were working possibly in tension with the advice above, but we would certainly be entitled to a kindergarten place. If we were not very good at 'pushing' for things for Adam, information about what is available would still have a high chance of reaching us, as would assistance in applying for support, but like others we would have to pay for our kindergarten place. At the kindergarten Adam would meet other young children (either with or without us being there) and we might draw on the services of our regional unit of the *Norwegian Support System for Special Education* for both advice and support regarding Adam's immediate progress and to assist in the assessment of his needs for support as he came into his local education system.

Educational services – 'special education' in 'schools for all'?

When the typical Norwegian primary school teacher looks across the faces of her about twenty-five pupils, approximately two to four of the children looking back have "special needs". Moreover, there are usually some other children who are at risk of formal identification. Teaching these pupils in regular education classrooms is a fact of life for all teachers in this country. The ideology of a school for all is clearly stated in Norwegian legislation and in the national curriculum . . . defined by equal formal access, by togetherness and by individually adapted teaching within the framework of a class.

(Moen 2004: 1)

The confidence shown by this author of a recent study of 'inclusion' in Norway's schools, that her description of a 'typical' class and all that follows holds good for most of Norway, is a common feature, as we have seen, of services in the two Scandinavian countries of our study. The fact that she then goes on to describe an, equally universal, *segregated* system having been in existence, reminds us of the issue of a paternalistic state being 'a good thing' if they 'do good' (i.e. adopt an approach in sympathy with what is perceived to be a 'values-led' basis) but 'a bad thing' if they 'impose' policies (e.g. sterilization) that the same perceivers regard as anathema to their values.

As long ago as 1881 Norway had a law on 'The Education of Abnormal Children' and thus the roots of a segregated special education system which lasted until the 1970s. Most people with more severe intellectual disabilities, as elsewhere, were described as 'ineducable'. Unlike some other places, however, the connection between normalization and inclusive education seems to have been stronger at that point and to have had a longer lasting effect. As the 1970s saw politicians regarding normalization and integration as the solution for those in institutions, so too, in education, 'integration' and then 'inclusion' became national policy. The old system still left a legacy, in that there is a perceived 'body of knowledge and expertise' of great significance to, and power in, the system of education for pupils with special needs, but their physical segregation, highlighted by normalization, became viewed as unacceptable. So the position in Norway, as viewed by a number of studies at the turn of the millennium (Meijer et al. 1997; Haug 2000) developed into one where inclusive education was strongly supported politically, although the system had elements of structure and power that could still support and even develop segregation within schools. Moen (2003) highlights the tension between the Education Act, and its allocation of extra resources for the education of pupils with special needs, and the labelling and segregating tendency inevitably attached to the process of ascertaining those pupils, also noting the likelihood of staff rooms being divided by whether teachers had taken the 'special education' option as part of their four-year training. The creation of the Norwegian Support System for Special Education also, of course defines an 'exclusive' group. This raises the notion, also noted in Sweden, of 'special education' within an inclusive system. Once a separate network of special schools was abandoned, compulsory education for all became the responsibility of the municipalities. As with other services, the bulk of resources come from the government through the national budget and local politicians have to distribute the scarce funds in compliance with legal requirements. A tension, as with LSS in Sweden, then comes between supposed 'rights' to services and the elasticity of individual authorities' budgets. 'High Schools', operating after the age of 16, are administered at county level, and though there is strong tendency for most pupils to move on to their local high school, there is again evidence of local variation in accommodating 'special needs' young people

(Moen and Gudmundsdottir 1997; Pettersson 2000; Flem et al. 2004). There appear to be very few private schools in Norway.

Mordal and Strømstad's (1998) overview below accords with the more informal accounts given to me by educational specialists on my visit to Trondheim:

> Generally, children must not be grouped according to ability, but such groupings may be used for short periods or for particular purposes, though not for the whole year. Exceptions can be made with parents' consent for children with special educational needs. Students continuously have their work corrected and commented upon, but no marks or examinations are given in primary schools. Secondary schools do have marks and a final exam, but students do not repeat years in either primary or in secondary schools . . .
>
> . . . In accordance with the Curriculum Guidelines, the school day is normally divided into lessons according to traditional academic subjects, such as Norwegian, mathematics, history, Christianity. The distinction between subjects is less explicit in primary school but very evident in secondary school . . . In addition to class teachers and subject teachers, most schools have special teachers and/or assistants assigned to teach pupils with special needs.
>
> (Mordal and Strømstad 1998: 103)

While we shall see far more variation, mixed motives, and mixed results in the application of inclusion in the remaining countries of this study, the vast bulk of evidence on Norway (Moen 2003; Flem et al. 2004; Haug 2004) indicates that, at the administrative and policy level at least, the same uniformity of response from the welfare state as in the de-institutionalization process has produced, from the education sector, a predominantly inclusive system. What does this mean in terms of the likely progress of a child with intellectual disabilities?

Mordal and Strømstad's (1998) translation of a contemporary White Paper concerning principles and guidelines for the new ten-year compulsory school gives the 'official' position. This defines an 'inclusive school' as a school where:

> Pupils with special needs shall participate equally in the social, academic and cultural community . . . all pupils – also those with special needs – as a general rule should go to school in their own district and get their education within the ordinary class . . . the teaching within the mixed ability class must be organised flexibly. Pupils can work in a variety of small and big groups or on their own. Such groups can also include pupils from other classes from the same or different grades.
>
> (Ministry of Education, Research and Church Affairs, 1995: 22–3)

This again accords with the impressionistic view of my visit, and is supported by the findings of Moen's study. The resources coming to schools in general as a result of the inclusion policy, and then with individual children as a result of formal assessment, provide the base on which so-called 'adapted education' can be applied *within* the physical environment of a mainstream school.

The description of Trondheim I was given is an example of inclusion in practice, and exceptions to it. The school system is part of one department of the municipality; the director covers education and social care for children and young people up to school leaving. A special school exists for autistic children, reflecting a common issue elsewhere, but otherwise special groupings, or simply individual placements, are provided for children with intellectual disabilities within the regular, local, school. Children are more likely to be taught in 'special' groups at the 13–16 age range, and even more so at 16–20/21, where they are usually in the 'practical' stream of 'High Schools' organized at county level. There appeared to be no other segregated education, so no equivalent, at least in Trondheim, of the Swedish 'training schools' for the most severely disabled. Preparation for post-school services is begun in advance, especially around 'work' possibilities, though as we shall see these can be limited as far as open employment is concerned. All of this is, of course, still largely dealt with by the municipality and the transition to adult services means a transfer within the local authority of known individuals, rather than a referral process to entirely different agencies, as in the non-Scandinavian countries of this book.

Physical integration in education is thus high in Norway, and compared to many, if not all, of the countries in our study, school provision for the majority of children with intellectual disabilities is attempting to be inclusive. Mordal and Strømstad (1998), in their review, still have questions. From an education system that many parents elsewhere on my tour, and others involved with the debates over inclusion, envied deeply, not least in terms of the assumption of responsibility of the local authority for all the children in its locality, these could be seen by some as a doctrine of perfectionism:

> Whether we use the terms 'integration', 'inclusion', 'adapted education' or 'one school for all', for any particular child we still have to ask: is this child really included as a full member of the school community, or have we only made superficial adaptations which leave the child just as isolated as in a special class or special school?
>
> (Mordal and Strømstad: 106)

My response to the above questions is partly revealed by the next box in 'Adam's World Tour', but it is also my perception, in both Sweden and Norway, that there is a greater emphasis within the school system on the *broad* development of individual pupils, including, importantly, relationships, and a lesser emphasis on narrowly academic achievement, and its concomitant competition on that basis between schools. Adaptation and inclusion therefore seem to be easier to achieve in the two Scandinavian countries than in societies where more appears to depend on quantifiable test or examination scores, in which pupils with intellectual disabilities will, by definition, appear at the lower end of the scale.

ADAM'S WORLD TOUR

Going to school in Norway

Adam's school experiences in Norway would be very similar to those in Sweden, though there might be more people with severe disabilities in his school. We, as his parents, would have been advised, by people involved up to his sixth birthday, to apply for Adam to be assessed for 'adapted education' by one of the regional advisory teams. This would normally generate resources for Adam to be in a regular class at his local primary school. Again like Sweden, we would expect there to be a local secondary school with a significant group of students with 'adapted education' programmes. Most schools would place Adam in a regular class, with some 'special group' work on particular subjects, though some have a separate 'special department' where he would be all the time. At high school level (16–19, though some people go on to 20 or 21), most young people with intellectual disabilities do the 'practical' routes, either in 'special' groups or with others, since not all high schools have 'special education' groups. Adam would be noted on the municipality's list of potential school leavers as he came up to 20 or 21, and plans would be made for his progression to day services. The words used to summarize his likely experience in Sweden apply exactly here, and so will be repeated.

Adam would therefore have gone through the school system alongside children with and without intellectual disabilities, though more frequently in the company of those on the 'special programme' route as he got older. The chance of his making friends, whose friendship went beyond and after school, would be significant, though more likely those friends would be other young people with intellectual disabilities.

Perhaps the conclusions of Moen (2004) are most appropriate to end this section, since they also link to a recurrent theme, that of the importance of the individual narrative of experience being set alongside and contributing to the larger theoretical and policy debate:

> School has been a hot topic in the public and political debates for years. New governments and a string of ministers apparently want to expose and emphasize their particular profile in educational politics. This leaves teachers to deal with the many and shifting educational directives that emerge. However, in spite of all the new ideas, the overarching vision for the Norwegian compulsory school seems to be firmly and deeply rooted. There appears to be agreement across established party lines that we should have an inclusive school for all our children in this country.
>
> (ibid.: 188)

Moen's study of teachers in Norway attempting to put the inclusion policy into effect, therefore concludes, among other things, that it is the values of the individual teachers, reinforced by or acting in contradiction to, an underlying ethos of the school, that really determine whether the answers to Mordal and Strømstad's questions are positive. My impression, from limited observation admittedly, is that for much of Norway they are certainly more positive than negative.

Into adulthood – daytime services

Given the age to which people are allowed to stay on at school in both Scandinavian countries, it is unsurprising that adult education immediately post-school is not very common. Though it has an entry in the overview of Table 3.1, therefore, we will not detail adult education as a separate section, since what use there is of such services seems to supplement the rest of what is available in the daytime. People will, as we have noted, already be 'on the books' of the adult services branch of the municipality and they may already have been channelled towards, or have some brief experiences of, the world of work. This is, however, rarely in what would be called 'open employment' since, as the 'first impact' story at the beginning of this chapter illustrates, supported by more rigorous studies (Seierstad 1998; Tøssebro and Lundeby 2002), the ability of the Norwegian system to deliver such an outcome is somewhat limited.

On the other hand, it would be true to say that the great majority of adults with intellectual disabilities in Norway are engaged in 'meaningful activities' and many of these would be defined by their content, if not their remuneration, as 'work'. The general principle, in both Scandinavian countries, is 'work-like' activities wherever possible, but through a combination of union agreements and perverse incentives through the benefit system 'open employment' in the sense of fully paid work in the competitive market, is scarce.

I visited a number of services in a small municipality near Trondheim, serving a total population of around 25,000, mostly in the central small town, but then spread thinly in rural communities. This gave what was described to me as a 'typical' range of both daytime and residential services. As we saw in the history section, even in the institutional times, so-called 'farming projects' were common in many of the rural parts of Norway. 'Work-based services', on farms, following the move from institutions, were therefore a natural 'community' equivalent, and are equally a part of contemporary services in many areas. The usual process seems to be that the municipality rent a certain part of a farm from the farmer (or, increasingly, a distant property owner) then use the farm for variety of occupational activities. The farm I visited carried out wood chopping/bagging (with some external contracts to sell the resultant product); all the activities involved with the keeping of chickens; and the maintenance of a semi-commercial vegetable and fruit garden. There were 15 people on the books, though usually only around ten attended at any one time, and not all attended for a full five days a week. There is no 'economic payment' as such, and this was, again, explained in terms of the adverse effects on benefits not making it worth more than 'pocket money' being awarded to individuals. The farm used to be on a regular bus route, but increasing use of rural properties by people as 'weekend cottages' has reduced the general demand for such services, so the municipality now has to organize transport specially for those working on the farm.

Norway has less of a specific statements of 'rights' to services than the LSS of Sweden, but there is a clear assumption that services, including day services, will be provided, and the policy is clearly work-oriented, except for those with the most severe multiple disabilities. In the small municipality, the farm project was part of a day service system which also had three day centres, plus a *snoezelen*-type complex (Wikipedia 2007) (though this was now shared with other groups). The full range of 'disability' categories is also covered in this municipality by a 'work centre' but I was informed that it is mostly used by groups other than people with intellectual disabilities. My informant, a person who had been in a senior position in services in the municipality for many years, said that there had been a few people over the years who had gone into open employment, and occasional 'work group' arrangements, as in Sweden, but these were limited because of the rurality of the municipality, disincentives to people (and their families) from the benefit system, and the general lack of a part of the service system specifically geared to finding people 'real work'. Most of this opinion was supported from other comments on my visit and from a number of the evaluation studies that accompanied the de-institutionalization process (Johansen and Kristiansen 2005; Tøssebro 2005) They conclude that day services have not changed as much as residential services. As we again have seen from the beginning of this chapter, when 'little institutions' were built as the first phase of the de-institutionalization process, those in need of 'daycare' i.e. therapeutic stimulation etc, still had it at the old institution. Others went to community-based, work-oriented day centres, sub-sidized but aiming to augment the subsidy with profit from production. These were what remained in the small municipality and, I was told, in many places in Norway. The one I visited was on a small industrial estate, and was part workshop and part post office for the estate. This latter part had a number of people working in the normal activities of a post office, but, again, they were not paid an economic wage. In the former part, the workshop, about six people were sitting around a table, making wrist muffs – the workshop also had a woodwork shop and loom. All the products were made to saleable qual-ity, though the economics of the centre did not appear to be its main control-ling force. Like the farm project, and like practice in many day services in Sweden, people did not attend the full five working days a week, especially those living in their own apartments, who are expected to spend one each week doing 'domestic duties' – cleaning, shopping, etc.

When the institutions fully closed, arrangements for people with severe and multiple disabilities seems to have been strongly influenced by the *snoeze-len* or multi-sensory centre. Even in a small municipality such as the one I visited, a full purpose-built centre, with all the different sensory rooms and multi stimulation technology had been constructed. It was staffed by two people with occupational therapy qualifications, who take referrals, conduct assessments and then organize a programme of sessions for individuals. This also involves instructing the various helpers who come with people, so that they can then run future sessions themselves. The centre was also part of a larger purpose-built building that has six bedrooms for 'short-term breaks' to which we will return when discussing residential services below, but as a part of day services it completes the range that we have outlined.

Residential services – homes for all?

The current position with regard to residential services in Norway still, to some extent, reflects the transition process from institutions, but as new people come into the system the trend towards fully integrated housing seems to be moving towards completion. As we noted, the law to close the large institutions also shifted the administrative responsibility to the municipality. This led, in the first instance, to many of the municipalities building smaller institutions and 'patriating' some people who were in institutions and wanted to stay in the institution area or had no links with their home area (Tøssebro 1996; Tøssebro and Lundeby 2002). These were often 'local' institutions of 50–60 people in 4–5 bedded units around central building with all the spe-cialists and offices, etc. The further reforms in the late 1980s and early 1990s, with the normalization/SRV training discussed by Kristiansen (1999) as its ideological drive, and with evaluation built in from beginning (Tøssebro 1992, 1996; Tideman and Tøssebro 2002) effectively said that small institutions were still institutions. Then came 'group homes' – individual apartments around a central common area – but these too, were still clearly 'service buildings' and thus did not meet the full SRV criteria. Then came blocks of apartments, blocks within broader groupings, and finally individual apartments. All but the last were built and provided by the municipalities, the last coming from ordinary apartments in the regular housing market. Given that municipalities can have a population ranging from 350 people to the millions of Oslo, there are very different issues depending on that size. As with Sweden, the central government allocation of funds to municipalities is on the basis of a formula from the centre, with social criteria such as the numbers of old people, rurality, etc., and then local politicians divide up the funding cake. Discussion with local politicians in both Scandinavian countries confirmed the views from elsewhere that there is not much flexibility in redirecting services because of the obligations to those already in existence, though initiatives from government can attract earmarked extra money. Reform of intellectual disability services, assumed to have been a 'success', is not now an earmarked area.

Because of this gradual move towards ordinary apartments, the more able seem to have gone first into, ironically, the most sheltered housing. Those with significant impairments were often the last to leave the 'mini-institutions', and by that time the ideology meant that they still were thought to be most beneficially placed in their own apartments (Saetersdal 1994; Tøssebro 2005). So a range of living, not directly related to ability, still exists, though the next generation, currently going through the regular school system, should be able to move out into their own apartments. A version of this state of affairs met me in the small municipality. As noted above, attached to the multi-sensory complex, and an integral part of the building design, was a six-bedroom residential building for 'short breaks' during individual weekdays or at weekends. I visited during the day on a weekday, and there were four people staying in the building. The three staff present consisted of some who had come with the people from their residences, while others were there all the time. 'Short breaks' appeared to be more common for young children than adults, who tend more often to be leaving home permanently.

Next door to the multi-sensory and respite building, ironically, was the first group home to be opened in the municipality. I was told that it was built originally for a woman from an institution ultimately deemed to be 'not intellectually disabled' but is now part of a row of four small apartments with various people with intellectual disabilities living there. These houses are also supported by staff from the multi-sensory building next door, and are about 50 yards, in the same building complex, from a three-storey block, where I was taken to visit a young man in his individual apartment. The overall complex was quite spread out, on the edge of the small town, with various other houses and apartments around, though the proportion of those for various vulnerable groups, elderly people, people with physical disabilities, made it a little bit of a 'service ghetto'. This was only to those who knew who the housing was for, however, since the visual image, apart from the multi-sensory unit, was of regular houses and apartments. The flat of the young man was similarly and comfortably ordinary, with a well-appointed and adequately spacious lounge, bedroom, and bathroom. He was home in the daytime because of a minor illness, affected by a degenerative condition, and, like the people in the 'group home', received support from workers from the nearby multi-sensory unit on a visiting basis. This would increase for this man as his condition deteriorated – there was no thought that this would force him to move from his apartment, at least in the near future.

'Non-direct' services

As with Sweden, financial benefits seem, in Norway, to be both a disincentive for fully competitive employment, and yet an incentive for parents to keep their offspring at home and use the respite system. They could, therefore, be said to militate against full inclusion in both residential and daytime activities. On the other hand, the role of NFU, in the same way as FUB, in adding to the momentum for de-institutionalization but not setting up services themselves, in contrast to many of the other countries in this book, has meant that NFU have continued to have an influence on policy without the vested interest that being a service provider often gives to parents organizations. Leisure activities, active group advocacy, and the provision of an information service to parents are thus all facilitated or provided by NFU. As a result, and this may be a broader point in relation to services largely organized and provided by the welfare states of Sweden and Norway, the issues of advocacy, self-advocacy and choice, so dominant in the remaining countries, appear to be less prominent. So we conclude this chapter with a similar account of Adam's potential life as a citizen of Norway to that which applied in Sweden, and an elusive notion of the difference between these two Scandinavian neighbours.

ADAM'S WORLD TOUR

An adult citizen of Norway

Our picture of Adam at school in Norway has already given the clue to what would happen to him at the age of 20 or 21. He would have already been noted on our municipality's list of school leavers and, at school, would probably have tried out a number of vocational type activities. If we were in one of the many rural areas in Norway, Adam might well be engaged in work on a farm project, or, if we made particular efforts as parents or had some sort of contact with the academic world, attempts might be made to get him the sort of open employment that was demonstrated by the young lady whose story started this chapter.

As he moved into his twenties, he would be offered the chance to move into his own apartment, probably on his own or with a person he had chosen to share with, though if we left it totally to the service system there would be some chance that he might be placed in an older 'group home' with two or three other people.

His social life would be assisted by NFU, if we wished to get involved, though this would probably have been set in train through his school experiences, as would personal friendships and potentially more serious relationships. As in Sweden, we as parents would still have a considerable say in what happened in this and other aspects of Adam's adult life, but if we took no interest the state would probably still provide both somewhere to live and some meaningful activity in the day.

The chapter opened with a sense of what this might be, based on the wartime experiences of occupation and collaboration, with their simultaneous tendency towards both a divided notion of nationalism and a concern for the incarcerated. The latter would lend weight to the anti-institution movement, but the former left me with a sense, difficult to explain, of a fine line between beneficent and malign authoritarianism, noted above in the specifically Norwegian experiences of the sterilization issue, and in the efficiency of de-institutionalization. As with all impressions, the generalizability of such thoughts may be of limited value, and it should be clear that my overall impression of Norwegian services is equally as positive as those of Sweden. As we move on to a country of similar size to these two Scandinavian welfare states, with services equally determined by central government, yet administered and delivered totally differently, my liberal reservations regarding Sweden and Norway may be put into a much more realistic context.

4 New Zealand
A values led market?

I wonder if I shall fall right through the earth! How funny it'll seem to come among the people that walk with their heads downwards! The Antipathies, I think – (she was rather glad no one was listening, this time, as it didn't sound at all the right word) – but I shall have to ask them what the name of the country is, you know. Please, Ma'am, is this New Zealand or Australia? . . . And what an ignorant little girl she'll think me! No, it'll never do to ask: perhaps I shall see it written somewhere.

(Lewis Carroll)

INSTANT IMPACTS

New Zealand – valued options; learning to drive or meeting the Prime Minister?

This story concerns a young man with Down's syndrome whom I met in Auckland. His mother, a senior person in a campaigning organization, showed me their latest newsletter, with a picture of her son, then aged 17, meeting the Prime Minister at an agency event. What quickly became clear, however, was that her son's choice of valued options went well beyond momentary connections in high places. Much of this came as a result of his being the subject of a relatively rare set-up in New Zealand, a so-called 'circle of friends'. The need for this arrangement had particularly arisen when the young man was beginning to experience difficulties at mainstream school, the first person with Down's syndrome at this particular establishment, though inclusion is not a rare phenomenon in New Zealand. Once the circle had been set up, however (with the formal title of a 'micro-board' which appears to have some significance because of the way services are delivered in New Zealand), they quickly got into wider issues than just his schooling. The benefit to the young man had many aspects, and the story of the 'micro-board' was not all plain sailing, but one key aspect that all agreed on was an increase in confidence, so that when he asked his father if he could learn to drive, the request was taken seriously. Currently still off-road in his learning, the probability of his joining the Auckland traffic is nevertheless high. As well as the specific issue of the driving, this story raises the more subtle differences between the countries in terms of the degree of activism by parents, and supporting and campaigning groups, to get services that they know exist, which are often trumpeted by governments and agencies as 'success stories', but which are often denied to the majority of people. So the question then becomes one of access to services, rather than ignorance or dispute about what represents quality.

Introduction: Aotearoa – New Zealand

> *E nga mana, e nga reo, e nga karanga maha o nga hau e wha tena koutou katoa.*
> *All people, all voices, all the many relations from the four winds.*

No one looking at intellectual disability in New Zealand can avoid the issue of history, and the place in the culture of the different ethnic groups who arrived in the islands over the centuries. Chapter 1 outlined, among other things, the much more recent arrival of the third group, named *pàkehà* by those they quickly outnumbered: the Màori, the *tangata whenua* or people of the land, and others from wider Pacific Islands. The arrival of these latter two groups, especially Pacific Islanders, is less clearly documented, though power-ful traditions put the time of the Màori arival at around a thousand years before the British, in *Waka* (long canoes) from Hawaiiki around 750 AD. Chapter 1 has also noted that the continuing presence of the Màori, and the nature of the colonizing process, have had a significant effect on the make-up of contemporary New Zealand society, especially in the past decade or so. Far more so than in the other British colonies or ex-colonies that are the subject of the next three chapters, the presence, and increasing power of, the descendants of those who met the whaling boats in the nineteenth century impinge on life in New Zealand in 2006. Developments seem to this outsider to be following an uneasy, but steady, path of cultural diversity, some degree of coming together in terms of the real meaning of the Treaty of Waitangi, but with a concomitant, paradoxical, degree of separateness. This process still has a way to go in playing itself out, but is significant enough to be discussed in a way that will not be the case in those other three countries.

The reason that we move on to New Zealand in our order of countries, however, has more to do with the *governance* of services than the real dif-ferences I perceived in how 'first peoples', including those with intellectual disabilities, are part of their respective societies. Unlike Australia, Canada, and the USA, and even the UK to a limited extent, local government in the first three countries of this book has few powers over the *overall* shape and financing of services, still less the ability, held by States or Provinces in Australia, Canada, and the USA, to set their own laws, raise their own taxes, and decide on their financial priorities, sometimes in conflict with their central governments. So New Zealand's policy on intellectual disability, like the LSS in Sweden or the closure policy in Norway, is definitely driven by the centre, and thus can be examined with a degree of consistency across the nation as a whole.

There, however, apart from a rough similarity in physical size and population spread, the congruence between the first three countries ends. As we shall see, central government policy in New Zealand is not implemented by the equivalent of the municipalities in Scandinavia, nor are the great majority of those involved in *direct* service provision employees of the government, local or national. Instead, New Zealand services are provided by independent agencies, many of whom are organizations originally set up by parents or parents' groups, and their eligibility to provide services is itself decided by independent agencies commissioned by the government. So in many ways we are going from the two examples of the Scandinavian welfare state to an out-and-out market of welfare, though it appears to be a market governed by statements of values and mission that the group of people who originated the principle of normalization in the late 1960s, and those who went on to promulgate Wolfensberger's formulations of SRV, would recognize.

Historical development of services – from *colonization* to segregation, normalization, Social Role Valorization, and beyond

Early developments – protection of her majesty

The Treaty of Waitangi, signed in 1840, giving the British Crown the power to govern the new settlers while giving 'her majesty Queen Victoria's protection' to them, but retaining Màori ownership of their lands, rivers, fisheries and forests, is an increasingly prominent feature of current New Zealand life. As we saw in Chapter 1, the introduction, in 1996, of a proportional representation voting system called MMP has meant that more Màori now have a voice in government and parliament, and the continued working of the Treaty of Waitangi Commission has resulted in a number of land claim settlements and other developments towards social, economic and educational initiatives based on Màori protocol and culture. Much of this could be considered reparation for the differential interpretation of the Treaty, most often in favour of the Crown, that typified its first 150 or more years.

In terms of services for people with intellectual disabilities, we can observe the continuing tendency for the influence of ideas from, first, the mother country, and then the 'western world' in general, to inform and even dominate policy and thinking (Millier 1999). In addition, continued migration, from the UK in particular, did not just mean that *ideas* were imported, but also people who were in positions to put them into effect. Thus a census, first introduced in the UK in 1801, was imported to New Zealand in the 1870s, as was the language used to describe the 'dependent groups' it discovered – 'deaf and dumb, blind, lunatics, idiots, epileptics, paralysed, and crippled and deformed'. The notion of 'public support for the poor' realized in England in the form of the 'workhouse' and the beginnings of 'public hospitals' was also imported, with a similar grouping together of people with intellectual disabilities among all the other recipients of 'poor relief' (Moore and Tennant 1997).

Hospital and charitable aid boards were in charge of these, providing income maintenance support as well as hospital and 'asylum' care, channelling funds from central and local government taxes to organizations, known as 'separate institutions'. The 'quasi-voluntary' nature of these institutional organizations also matched the parallel growth, in late Victorian England, of 'charities', often with a religious basis, that gave opportunities for the wealthier members of society to attempt to deal with the 'problem of the poor'. The paternalism and division of these organizations into 'deserving' and 'undeserving' recipients of their services (as well as their policy, that continued well into the twentieth century, of shipping off orphaned and/or illegitimate children to the colonies) has been well documented (Bagnell 1980; Bean and Melville 1983) as has their link to the eugenics movement.

The twentieth century – eugenics and institutions

The growth of science, especially medicine, as a 'solution' to social ills, was therefore no stranger to the colonies on the other side of the globe, and when a young Scotsman was recruited by the Mental Hospitals Department in New Zealand in 1911, the idea of separate hospitals, or asylums, for specific groupings of people was also well established. Theodore Gray provides an interesting case study in the import of both ideas and people that fitted well with the confident and established Anglo-centric ruling classes of New Zealand at the turn of the century (Brunton 2006).

Gray was born in Aberdeen and graduated in medicine from the University in 1906. After a short period in general practice, he went to work at Kingseat Asylum, Newmachar, Scotland, the first British psychiatric hospital built entirely of villas that segregated patients according to diagnosis, behaviour, dependency and gender; more benevolent, at least in principle, than some of the 'bedlams' of the south of England. Gray was later to foster this system in

New Zealand, and to give the name Kingseat to a new hospital at Papakura. After his arrival in 1911, Gray had served, in quick succession, at Porirua Mental Hospital, Auckland Mental Hospital, and Seacliff Mental Hospital, near Dunedin, and after the war, in 1921, became medical superintendent of Nelson Mental Hospital, which he planned to replace with a 'villa hospital' at Stoke. Four years later, the acting inspector general of mental defectives, considering Gray a promising administrator, appointed him to the post of acting medical superintendent of the Auckland Mental Hospital and shortly afterwards deputy inspector general of mental defectives. Gray succeeded his patron as permanent head of the Mental Hospitals Department in 1927. By this time, of course, the Mental Deficiency Act of 1913 in the UK was in full swing, with a large building programme of the ironically named 'colonies', generally by adding 'villas' to the existing Victorian asylums to expand capacity and carry out the segregative eugenically based policies of the Act's originators. It also had, in the category of 'moral defective' a classification not included in New Zealand's 1911 Act, but which was a key part of the eugenicists' case. It is no surprise therefore that New Zealand had its own Inquiry into Mental Defectives and Sexual Offenders in 1924, to which Gray gave evidence. The title of the inquiry gives a clue as to its tone, and the submissions to it, including Gray's, contained the customary presentation of intellectual disability as evidence of 'degeneracy' of the population, and thus a threat to national efficiency. The need to prevent the procreation of the unfit was a major theme in the Committee's recommendations, though it took four years for draft legislation to be prepared. Meanwhile Gray was undertaking an overseas study tour prior to assuming his leadership role in 1927, reinforcing his solidly eugenicist views with experiences from Europe. Some of the resultant recommendations in a report of the tour were included in the Mental Defectives Amendment Bill of 1928. Gray proposed, with no obvious ironic intent, separate 'farm colonies' for people with intellectual disabilities, as well as statutory registration, psychological screening clinics, and sterilization. Sterilization was part of the more controversial details dropped in subsequent legislation, however, and, as his biographer notes, the mood was changing in certain countries on the more radical outcomes of eugenics. 'Gray subsequently stayed silent about his views on eugenics and the sterilisation of the mentally unfit, and on his chairmanship of the short-lived Eugenics Board' (Brunton 2006).

Whatever the extent of sterilization, the institutions were firmly in place, increasingly being 'medicalized', but, as in the UK, not part of the mainstream hospital system until after the Second World War. Gray's career continued, and his biographer's notes on his preferences and power in the system until the Second World War give a familiar picture to the other countries of this study, especially the imperial centre, Britain, that still had many of those countries as 'colonies' of its own (Brunton 2006).

A *pàkehà* service – low take-up by Màori

The increasing medicalization of disability services in general, and the 'colonies' in particular, figures in a study of the very low use of services by Màori. At a philosophical level it contrasts the technical and medical focus on the physical body (including the mind), which *pàkehà* health professionals espoused, with Màori views on 'well-being'. 'It is likely that Màori had different perceptions of just what was (and is) a "disability" ' (Moore and Tennant 1997: 12). A further issue, namely the separation, that came with institutionalization, from *whànau* (family grouping) and other traditional supports, is then raised. 'Most services, public and non-public were monocultural in emphasis, and those limited numbers of Màori who used such services probably did so at a cost to their cultural identity and *whànau* links' (ibid.: 12).

The 1950s and 1960s – medicalization and the growth of IHC

Gray's life illustrates New Zealand's fit with the institutions that predominated in the 'western world', including the 'old' (euphemism for white) part of the 'Commonwealth of Nations', that still maintained major economic, social and intellectual bonds between countries of the British Empire, as its political power began to decline after the Second World War.

New Zealand's relative prosperity, indeed, owed a great deal to Commonwealth markets, especially in the mother country, so it is not surprising that the model of 'care' in intellectual disability which emerged in the UK with the setting up of the National Health Service should have been followed in the colonies. In New Zealand, the 'mental health system', including many of the quasi-voluntary institutions such as Templeton Farm in Christchurch, opened in 1929 for 'high-grade imbeciles and low-grade feeble-minded cases without psychotic complications', merged with the main health departments. Like the UK, where the institutions for intellectual disability were very much at the bottom of the pecking order within the NHS (Race 2002b), the existing New Zealand facilities changed very little with the advent of their new administrative arrangements (Capie 1997). In another parallel with the home country and others in this book, a pressure group of parents then grew up from those dissatisfied with conditions in which their children were living. The Intellectually Handicapped Children's Society (IHC) was formed in 1949. Unlike its UK counterpart, however, until much later, IHC went beyond lobbying and into significant service provision. In 1953, it began to acquire properties for short-stay homes and occupational groups. Still largely focusing on children, IHC benefited from amendments to the Mental Health Act in 1954 and 1956, which made it easier for the association to run short-stay homes, and from increasing approval by the Minister of Health for limited capitation subsidies and grants for capital expenditure. Demands on the 'radical' services of IHC seem then to have increased (Moore and Tennant 1997), although few studies, even the official 'histories' of IHC and other agencies such as the Crippled Children's Society (an earlier formed agency, originally providing care for children with physical disabilities, but also taking some with intellectual disabilities) claim that their service provision was radically different to the institutions (Carey 1960; Millen 1999). What they did have was the cachet, referred to above, of the 'voluntary agency' and by calling their residential establishments 'hostels' or 'farms' or 'residential schools' they, perhaps unconsciously, moved a small distance from the medical orientation of the hospital. On the occupational side, IHC's centres gained a boost, along with similar provision for other disabled groups, with the passing of the Disabled Persons Employment Promotion Act in 1960. This exempted operators of sheltered workshops from the level of employment standards required elsewhere, thus creating the situation, as we have already seen in the Scandinavian countries, where there was a distinction between 'sheltered employment' and employment in the open market.

Growth in this area within IHC added to their increasing residential provision, but was somewhat uneasily combined with campaigning for rights in education and a growing critique of the institutions. IHC had been in touch with the embryonic movement around normalization, and sent key individuals overseas to observe and report (Hartnett 1997). Perhaps the most prominent of these, Dr Donald Beasley, made a Nirje paper on normalization compulsory reading in a 1971 course taught to IHC staff and that year also saw publication of the first locally written papers on normalization (Capie 1997). As we saw in Chapter 1, New Zealand has a relatively small population and geographical area, and when this is combined with the fact that, in all countries studied and probably universally, the world of intellectual disability is a small one, contact between people and sharing of information is, then as now, that much easier. Thus the broad principles were widely disseminated, strengthening IHC's position as the 'radical' voice throughout the country. Wolfensberger's (1972) formulation of normalization began to be taught in IHC's in-service training courses from the late 1970s, and in 1979 the IHC officially adopted the principle of normalization in its Philosophy and Policy Document (Mitchell and Mitchell 1985). Residential Standards, known as 'The Blue Book', incorporating elements of normalization and the evaluation tool PASS (Wolfensberger and Glenn 1975), were devised as guidelines and a training tool for IHC staff (New Zealand Institute on Mental Retardation 1980; Capie 1997).

In New Zealand, therefore, as well as commitment and leadership generated by training, a developing *evaluation* process appears to have been significant. A separate agency, Standards and Monitoring Services Trust (SAMS), was later set up by IHC in conjunction with the Department of Social Welfare, and was influential, along with broader social policy events in the

1990s, in developments that led to the current New Zealand Disability Strategy.

Before that, however, the other side of the growth of IHC needs to be considered. Alongside the national organization's espousal of normalization had come, sometimes from outside and sometimes at local level from within, dissent over the IHC's role. Moore and Tennant (1997) describe issues regarding IHC's size, its decision in the late 1980s to abandon large hostels, jealousy from smaller organizations, and a feeling of loss of autonomy by local IHC groups. What was to come next, however, as New Zealand moved into the 1990s, certainly saw a continuing role for IHC, but also saw wider social policy issues begin to have a dramatic effect on the service system itself.

The 1990s – the welfare market cometh

The experiences of reforms in intellectual disability services noted in the two Scandinavian countries took place within stable welfare states, and thus could be very specific to intellectual disability. We will more often find, in the other five countries, including New Zealand, intellectual disability services being swept up in a whirlwind of change to welfare services overall, themselves only part of changes in the financing and administration of public services in general. As we shall see later in this chapter, specific policy documents on intellectual disability did emerge after the turn of the millennium in New Zealand and the UK, but these were both in the context of a new general social welfare environment that the 1990s brought about.

In New Zealand, as in England, the seeds of these more general changes had already been present in the 1980s. The downturn in world economies of that decade had been particularly felt in New Zealand, adding to the earlier economic blow to preferred trade caused by its largest traditional market, the UK, joining the European Economic Community (now the European Union) in 1973 (Castles et al. 1996). Policy analysts, Castles and Shirley (1996) note the extensive changes brought in by the New Zealand Labour governments of 1984–90, with the underlying aim of allowing the free play of market forces in the economy, removing what were seen as 'bureaucratic' regulations and subsidies that typified previous government policies towards the economy and the welfare state. Rather sooner than many countries, including even the mother country, New Zealand undertook a vigorous programme of social reforms (Holmes and Wileman 1995). The effect of these reforms on intellectual disability services was not, initially, that great, in that many institutions still remained under direct government control, and there already existed, in IHC in particular, agencies, outside of direct government employ, providing services. Following Labour's re-election in 1987, however, the quest for greater efficiency in government – contrasted with the assumed market-driven efficiency in the private sector – led to legislation which significantly changed the governance of the public service, the 1988 State Sector Act. Space does not permit a full account of the details, but the essence of the legislation was to change the notion of a 'career civil servant', moving up the ranks and often changing ministries but essentially part of the government machinery, to an employee of an 'agency', headed by a 'Chief Executive' and measured by a series of 'performance targets'. This was then further bolstered, in its resource implications, by the Public Finance Act of 1989.

The National Party government, elected in 1990, to the right of the Labour Party, was emboldened to go further with the move to a market of welfare, particularly in the area of health. What became known as the 'Health Service reforms' were begun in 1991, and moved considerably further away from 'state welfare' than similar changes being implemented in the UK after the Conservative government's 1990 NHS and Community Care Act.

As far as intellectual disability services were concerned, the historic role of organizations like IHC again meant that they could use their 'independent' status to bid for funding under the new arrangements that separated 'purchasers and providers' of services. The actual services on the ground differed relatively little from what had gone before, though the normalization and SRV influence, especially through visits by Michael Kendrick and others from the USA (Millier 1999) was making inroads into the service system in both traditional agencies like IHC and CCS, but also in the increasing number of newer, smaller, agencies that would emerge under the welfare reforms.

Set alongside this, however, were two other factors that modified the broader changes to some extent and could be said to have led to the context for, and essence of, the New Zealand Disability Strategy of 2001. They also have wider implications for the remaining countries in this book, and thus will be dealt with, as we did with the first appearance of the broader issue of eugenics, at slightly greater generality and length in this chapter, with briefer reference in later chapters.

The influence of the social model of disability

The first of the two factors has been alluded to, but only briefly, in the previous two chapters. Its particular significance in the different countries, as far as intellectual disability is concerned, reflects, in my view, its different origins in those countries and the relationship of its originators with the movements and networks around normalization and SRV. I have, with others (Race 1999; Race et al. 2005) addressed elsewhere the issue of the growth of the so-called 'social model' or 'social theory' of disability in the UK, and its connection with normalization/SRV and the development of intellectual disability services. Readers unfamiliar with those debates will find, if they consult the literature, something of a clash between adherents of the social model, usually from what has become known as the 'disability studies' area of academia, and those involved with the normalization/SRV networks, whose main roots are in intellectual disability (Race 2002c; Barnes et al. 2002). In examining the different countries of this book, however, it was fascinating to compare the greater ease with which those involved in 'disability studies' in Scandinavia could accommodate *both* the social model and normalization/SRV. This contrasted with, especially, the UK, where from a position of mutual ignorance, in the true sense of that word, exemplified by the debate between Oliver and Wolfensberger at the Ottawa conference of 1994 (Flynn and Lemay 1999), there grew two hostile camps, and a virtual academic apartheid for a number of years.

New Zealand appears to have gone, in the context of ideas at least, more in parallel with Scandinavia than the mother country, in that normalization/SRV and the social model can at least be discussed in the same breath, and be held as ideas in common by some people. This may be because common ground was forged, to some extent, in opposition to the welfare reforms of the 1990s, and reflected in the key fact that the New Zealand Disability Strategy of 2001 covers *all* disabled groups, with an important role for intellectual disability. We shall see in later chapters that the position in Australia and Canada also appears to be somewhere in between Scandinavia and the UK, though social model adherents, especially in Australia, did have a significant period of hostility to normalization/SRV. The USA, as we shall see in its own chapter, is extremely difficult to summarize, having such a wide range of views and services.

In their chapter of a New Zealand-based book with authors from both the social model and normalization/SRV, Munford and Sullivan (1997) note that the key issue in the disability world over the health reforms had changed from debate over which *organization* should administer services, to the fact that the actual service *system* was being framed as a market, reflected in the Health and Disability Services Act of 1993. The notion, from the social model, of a united voice for all disabled people taking political action against medical model adherents and government legislators, could therefore also include a broader political opposition to the market reforms. Campaigners within the intellectual disability world were part of this broader opposition, which seems to have overshadowed the more arcane academic debate between the social model adherents and the normalization/SRV networks that dominated elsewhere.

Into the third millennium – markets and managers

The second more general factor affecting intellectual disability services in New Zealand that also applies to other countries concerns what has been called 'managerialism'. Many observers claim it stems from, and is an inevitable outcome of, the marketization of welfare (Raper 2000; DiNitto and Cummins 2004). Certainly, to continue the New Zealand story, the playing out of political and social policy changes after the perceived 'failure' of the health reforms lends weight to the thesis that whatever the position of governments on the old 'left–right' spectrum, managerialism still emerges. Victory in 1999, to a coalition of the Labour Party and the Alliance Party, a grouping of smaller parties including the 'New Labour' Party and the Green Party, changed political power, but not, many would argue (Cheyne et al., 2000) the continued development of significant change in the *culture* by which services of all kinds were managed. Discussion of this phenomenon begins with the issue of '*style over substance*'. Like Tony Blair's 'New Labour' victory in the UK in 1997, the coming to power of a left of centre coalition in New Zealand did not produce a fundamental change from the market system that underlay the provision of welfare, or most other government services, let alone any notion of the taking back into public ownership services that had been completely privatized in the neo-liberal economic period. Instead, again like Blair's Labour Party, a great deal of attention was paid by the new coalition to 'presentation of government policy' and 'listening' to the people, via 'reference groups', 'strategy groups' and other consultation bodies. As noted, many commentators are of the view that the style and culture of management are dependent upon the form of organization, in particular, whether such organizations are operating in a competitive market, or whether their survival is not dependent on beating the competition, but on maintaining the political support of their 'patrons', or commissioners, especially if such patrons are governments (Enteman 1993; Rees and Rodley 1995; Clarke et al. 2000). One of the key debates, noted by Munford and Sullivan (1997) above, that was raised in the 1990s in particular, as the full force of marketization moved from industrial and utility services to education and welfare services, is the difficulty of applying doctrines that relate to *consumers*, in the sense of those who have a free choice to purchase or otherwise, to people who *need services*, the absence of which could, in some cases, be fatal. What I think is agreed, and I heard this from many contacts on my trip as well as, for at least ten years, experiencing its effects in my work and reading about it in the literature, is that the key difference in the culture of management that goes under the name of 'managerialism' covers the *knowledge* and *connection* between the managers of service organizations and the people who use the services. As we have seen in the previous two chapters, however, what counts as 'knowledge', or 'expertise' and its *power* over what happens in services, can be problematic. In those chapters, and in the historical part of every chapter on the individual countries, we come across the role played by 'knowledge', in the form of the views of whichever professional group held sway at any particular point in time. First, from the broad 'medical' world, then the psychologists, with their brave new worlds of testing, behaviourism and psychoanalysis, all mixed up among the eugenicists, knowledgable or merely excitable about the degeneration of the race. In terms of the allocation of resources and the *management* of the institutions, however, the 'experts' held sway by their professional authority, not their expertise in management. Only when the assumption that the 'efficiency of industry' was needed in the new welfare markets did the notion come into effect that: (1) costs of welfare should be taken down to the level of detail of an industrial concern, particularly the ability to connect them to individual recipients wherever possible, to allow for full or partial private payment; and (2) that the *measurement* of costs and benefits was possible in welfare services, thus developing the industrial notion of 'value for money' and 'return on investment' into services for people. Thus follows the idea that the expertise required to determine what should happen in services is that of a generic 'strategic manager' of resources, manipulating costs and benefits so as to, in the commonly heard phrase, 'achieve the objectives within existing budgets'. What I have personally observed over this period, and saw on my visits, is a change to a situation where those responsible for the *commissioning* of services are increasingly people who know very little about intellectual disability. Where this was not the case, I found an increasing frustration that what seemed to count in the career prospects of those responsible for administering resources was not stories of success with individual people or services, nor even a generalized sense of development. Instead, success is now measured in terms of meeting targets, defined arbitrarily in very broad terms, usually those which can be quantified, but, most importantly, within decreasing financial limits. It is, of course, a corrolary of the greater 'freedom' of the market place that taxation, and therefore public spending, are kept to a minimum, and thus the countries who have gone along the so-called 'neoclassical' economic route have also sought to 'roll back the state'. This places those in charge of state welfare spending, whether directly as managers of their own services or as commissioners of agency provided services, increasingly in a position of being rationers of welfare.

As we move to what follows from this historical section, namely the New Zealand Disability Strategy of 2001 (Minister for Disability Issues 2001), we shall therefore see, as we will in the countries of the rest of the book, some fine rhetoric about the 'vision' of services, and national or regional 'strategies' based on similar sets of 'key principles'. Unlike the two Scandinavian countries, however, there will be much less *specific* definitions of good practice, or of people *allocating* the resources having a specific background in intellectual disability.

Services in New Zealand – an impression

A 'long-term plan for changing New Zealand from a disabling to an inclusive society'?

Though it has, in common with LSS in Sweden, the combination of a clearly laid out policy and the likelihood of relatively uniform applicability throughout the regions of the country, the New Zealand Disability Strategy (Minister of Disability Issues 2001, hereafter NZDS) differs from LSS in two key areas, which connect with the two issues discussed at the end of the history section above. The first is that the NZDS document covers all disabled groups, whereas LSS is specifically concerned with, in the English translation, 'mental impairment'. The second difference is that the NZDS is not a law, and is framed in terms of 'objectives', a similar situation to that which we will see in Chapter 8, on English services. This is significant, not only in the light of the previous section on managerialism, but also in the fact that *entitlement* to *specific services* is not contained in the NZDS. This means that its objectives can be met in a number of ways, and it becomes a matter of interpretation whether, for example, the government is succeeding in objective 8, 'support quality living in the community for disabled people'; a somewhat harder task than being able to tell whether a person in Sweden has a 'Residence with special services for adults or other specially adapted housing'. It is also, being a law rather than a 'strategy', an easier task to use LSS to ensure that the entitlement is carried out.

Nevertheless, compared with a number of countries in this book, the NZDS at least represents, in my view, a public, and nationwide, commitment to meeting the sort of goals for disabled people that stem from both normalization/ SRV and the social model of disability, and also, importantly, specifically acknowledges disability issues in relation to Màori and Pacific Island people. This will be examined below, but first we present the normal overview of services in New Zealand in Table 4.1.

Pre-natal services – a 'haphazard' middle way?

In its only reference to pre-natal screening and disability that I can discover, the NZDS Objective 1, 'Encourage and educate for a non-disabling society' has, under 'Actions1.4', the following statement – 'Include the perspectives of disabled people in ethical and bioethical debates.' Perhaps the following 'Action', number 1.5, which promises to 'Encourage ongoing debate on disability issues' could also be said to be related to pre-natal screening, since it is clearly a 'disability issue' as well as an 'ethical and biological debate'.

A number of writers have argued that the influence of the social model on the issue of screening has been less successful in terms of the model's stated goal of valuing difference than it has been on achieving change in other disability issues (Morris 1991; Shakespeare 2006). On abortion in general, New Zealand's laws are put firmly in the middle of the worldwide range of 'liberality' devised by the US-based pro-abortion pressure group, the Center for Reproductive Rights (CRR 2005), and, to judge from a recent report prepared for the New Zealand Ministry of Health, there appears to be a relatively low amount of screening going on, again mainly for the over-35s. According

Table 4.1 Schematic overview of 'services' that affect the lives of people with intellectual disabilities in New Zealand

'Service'	Formal organizational place	Specialist or generic?	Main source(s) of funding*
Pre-natal services	District Health Boards General Practitioners Family Planning Clinics	Generic and specialist	Taxation, via Ministry of Health (Clinical Services and Disability Services)
Post-natal and early childhood services	District Health Boards. Early childhood agencies, some voluntary	Generic clinical services, but agency input varying in specialization	Taxation, via Ministry of Child Youth and Family for generic services and Ministry of Health (Clinical Services and Disability Services) for specialist – grants and direct funding of agencies, payments for individual children.
Non-educational services for children	Agencies, including those providing 'out of family care'	Specialist and generic	Taxation via Ministry of Health (Disability Services) – grants and direct funding of agencies, payments for individual children
Education services – children and young adults	Local School Boards	Generic and specialist	Taxation, derogated to Local School Boards for generic services, plus various special education funding streams
Education services – adults	Polytechnics and colleges	Generic and specialist	General tertiary education funding plus Special Supplementary Grant
Residential services – adults	District Health Boards Agencies Housing New Zealand Corporation	Generic and specialist	Taxation, administered through Ministry of Health (Disability Services)
Daytime services – non-work	Agencies	Largely specialist	Taxation, administered through Ministry of Health (Disability Services)
Daytime services – work	Agencies, especially Workbridge	Largely specialist	Taxation, administered through Ministry of Social Development (Work and Income) State Services Commission Mainstream Programme

Leisure assistance	Agencies	Specialist and generic	Taxation, administered through Sport and Recreation NZ, Creative NZ and Territorial local authorities
Advocacy services	Agencies	Specialist	Taxation, administered through Ministry of Health (Disability Services)
Financial Assistance	Ministry of Social Development (Work and Income)	Specialist within generic service	Taxation, administered through Ministry of Social Development (Work and Income)
Parental 'support services'	Acting as all parents – not a job in an organization, but can be active in agencies. Many agencies originally parent groups, especially IHC	Specialist, in that all children are different	Own finances

Note: Where the intellectual impairment is caused by an accident in childhood, including around birth, some of these services may be funded through the Accident Compensation Corporation (ACC).

to the report, screening practice had developed haphazardly with little co-ordination and no quality control. There was also no control over funding for screening, no idea how much screening costs, no guidelines for follow-up after a positive test and no agreement on what constituted a positive test (Stone and Austin 2004).

This concurs to a degree with the more personal accounts I received in two meetings on my visit to New Zealand, one with a parent support group, and one a more mixed voluntary group, called *Te Whānau Kotahi* (loosely translated as 'The all-embracing family'). The latter group included, and was formed as, an information and support group for parents, but also has an active membership of midwives, health visitors and other professionals involved in the birth of disabled children. In both of these groups, stories predominated of pressure being put on more women than just the over-35 age group, and certainly pressure for termination if disability was discovered. Whatever the true situation, the higher profile of disability brought about by the NZDS does at least seem to have allowed questions to be raised about the basic assumption of the undesirability of the birth of a disabled child.

Like many countries, New Zealand's abortion legislation dates back to the 1970s. The Contraception, Sterilisation, and Abortion Act 1977 (CS&A) set up the Abortion Supervisory Committee which reports annually to Parliament. Grounds for an abortion are contained in an earlier Act, the Crimes Act 1961 (as amended in 1977 and 1978), namely:

- serious danger to life;
- serious danger to physical health;
- serious danger to mental health;
- any form of incest or sexual relations with a guardian;
- mental subnormality;
- foetal abnormality (added in the July 1978 amendment).

Other factors which are not grounds in themselves but which may be taken into account are extremes of age, and sexual violation (previously rape). The CS&A Act also caused various other Acts affected by the legislation to be amended, including the Guardianship Act, whereby a female of any age may consent to or refuse an abortion, then implying that even a girl under 16 years cannot be forced by her parents to terminate or otherwise. In 2004, this section of the Guardianship Act was transferred to the Care of Children Act. The implications for the assumption of screening and abortion on discovery are clear, but actual practice, as the Stone and Austin (2004) report noted, is much more mixed.

'Initial' services – ACC, NASC and the beginning of agency involvement

At my meeting with the *Te Whànau Kotahi* group I also had the pleasure of meeting a young Pacific Island mother, who had sat with her young baby daughter, some few months old, at the back of the audience during my presentation. In talking to her afterwards, I was struck by the different possible outcomes: (1) for the woman and her daughter as Pacific Island people; and (2) for her as a mother who had just been awarded partial funding for her daughter's disability through the Accident Compensation Corporation (ACC).

The effect of the first of the factors, to my Western outsider's eyes, was the obvious support from her extended family for the young woman to look after a child with severe impairments. From my Western 'liberal' perspective, however, the strict hierarchy and belief regarding the lower status of both the mother and child that appears to be the situation of both women and disabled people in the Pacific peoples' culture, which also emerges clearly from the findings of the major survey that followed the NZDS (NHC 2003), were a problem. The NZDS does at least raise the issue publicly, and the 'Actions' under Objective 12, 'Promote participation of disabled Pacific peoples' (Minister for Disability Issues 2001) tacitly acknowledge a process of mutual learning, exemplified by the attendance of the young woman at what was, in fact, her first meeting with the *Te Whànau Kotahi* group.

On the second point, funding from the ACC can be used, as the note in

Table 4.1 explains, to pay for the provision of most services for people with disabilities. I was already aware of a perceived 'class distinction' between people who were able to access this money and those who were not, and the key issue regarding ACC can be deduced from the first two words of its name. The *Accident Compensation* Corporation, (my emphasis) is therefore *not* concerned with conditions, such as Down's syndrome, whose *causes* are unknown but occur during pregnancy, and are not deemed to be the result of 'personal injury' or 'accident'. ACC was set up by the Injury Prevention, Rehabilitation and Compensation Act 2001, as a so-called 'no-fault' compensation scheme, funded through social insurance and administered by the quasi-independent agency which represents the *Corporation* part of the name. Success in getting funding from the ACC for a disabled person depends crucially on that person's impairment being judged to have arisen from a 'personal injury' and is awarded to cover *only* the implications of that injury in terms of defined 'needs', following a lengthy and rigorous assessment process. An ACC case manager then works with, depending on the individual circumstances and point in life at which the personal injury occurs, the claimant, the family, perhaps employers, schools, and treatment providers, to determine what is defined as 'the most financially responsible solution from the identified options'. The point of causation is crucial here, especially with the significant number of people whose children's intellectual impairment is caused at or around birth. If, as was claimed for the lady I met, some aspect of the impairment can be attributed to hereditary genetic factors, then even if there was an acknowledged 'medical misadventure' at birth, the claimant may only get a partial payment. It does not take much imagination to realize the competing pressures of budgets, the uncertainty of causation of much of intellectual impairment, and the difficulty of separating one aspect of a child's impairment from another. It is also easy to imagine the tension between parents of two almost identical children, in terms of their presenting needs, one of whose needs were deemed to arise from a 'genetic cause' and the other an 'accident in the womb'. That being said, at least acceptance by ACC provides a legal entitlement to funding that is not often present in the more usual process of obtaining funding for services, the other set of initials, NASC.

Begun around the time of the National Government coalition of 1996, the Needs Assessment Service Co-ordination (NASC) system sought to go further, in the process of service commissioning, than many of its counterparts in other countries. It not only continued the split between purchasers and providers of services begun in the Health Reforms of the early 1990s, but also allocated the *commissioning* side of the equation to non-governmental organizations. At the time of my visit there were 11 such agencies, covering different regions of New Zealand, a small reduction from earlier numbers. As we have discussed above, the time when NASCs were set up seems to have been the high point of influence of normalization/SRV and the social model in New Zealand, and a number of key individuals with a significant background in intellectual disability (many originally involved with IHC) were part of the deliberations around the concept. NASC goes well beyond the assessment for early childhood services, with its main work covering assessment and arrangement of services for adults, but is important to consider the process at this stage of our thinking about New Zealand services as it is likely to be the first point of contact for many families with the system by which those services are administered. Put simply, NASCs are commissioned by the Ministry of Health to assess an individual's support needs, devise with them an appropriate service or group of services to meet those needs, and recommend to the Ministry the release of financial resources to fund the package. As one of the key individuals mentioned above, Lorna Sullivan describes the original concept, as the context for a critique of developments since that point:

> The concept from which NASC began to emerge was a concept of individual needs assessment and the active attempt by a service coordinator to secure as responsive a package of services as possible to address the needs identified by the disabled person and their family.
> This concept was not without its dilemmas, but was fundamentally simple and was based upon a belief that disabled people and their families could be trusted both to define their own needs and to work in a collaborative arrangement with the assessor to determine how best available resource might be spent on their behalf. To be successful an assessor would be a person with considerable experience in the lived experience of disability or in the delivery of disability support services and would have the ability to use all means at their disposal to set up flexible and responsive solutions that would make sense to the person using the service and be affordable within the prescribed financial limitations.
>
> (Sullivan 2001: 2)

Sullivan's critique partly relates to the managerialism issue, and refers to a 'shift in who has become the powerful master in this process'. She goes on to assert that 'NASC was established as a process to facilitate access to services for disabled people. It has now, in a very short period of 3–4 years, become a gatekeeper to limited resources' (ibid.: 2).

Five years after Sullivan's remarks I observed, in all the remaining countries of this book, similar processes. Whether it was commissioners directly employed by national, regional or local governments, or those, like New Zealand NASCs, contracted to commission services, tensions between their role to develop responsive packages of services for individuals, progressive practices in the field in general and the dead hand of bureaucratic budgets, seemed to be resolved, with notable but relatively few exceptions, by gate-keeping emerging as the dominant process. With that process there also appears, in many countries including New Zealand, to have been a complementary move towards standardization of assessment, in the sense that commissioning increasingly seems to involve fitting people into a series of standardized profiles, along with which goes a standardized package of services, which has to fit a diminishing budget. This then ties in with the increasing tendency to believe that people who manage such commissioning processes do not need to fit Sullivan's criteria for the early NASC advisors – 'a person with considerable experience in the lived experience of disability or in the delivery of disability support services' (ibid.: 2).

We are, of course, back to managerialism again, and the overwhelming impression from New Zealand, and the remaining countries, remains that it is a powerful force in preventing the sort of services and societies envisaged in documents like the NZDS from coming to greater fruition. As we go through the age and service range in New Zealand, this issue will recur.

Post-natal, early childhood, and non-educational services for children

My pun on the word 'initial' has resulted in a digression, though an important one, from impressions of the early contact of parents of intellectually disabled children with the New Zealand service system. Basic services available to *all* parents in New Zealand around the birth of a child, as elsewhere, revolve around health development and early detection of issues not apparent at birth. As noted, this does clash, to some extent, with the more holistic approach to child rearing of the Màori *whànau* and the Pacific peoples' extended family and kinship systems, especially in the identification of those falling within less clear-cut categorizations of intellectual disability. In practice, this may mean that those from Màori and Pacific Island communities with less obvious intellectual disabilities will not be 'identified' as early as others from the majority *pàkehà* families, perhaps not an entirely unmixed blessing. For those with more obvious conditions, such as Down's syndrome, or those with multiple disabilities, then the system of visiting from health professionals in the early years seems to be reasonably consistent. What then becomes an issue, however, is payment for, and access to services, via the systems discussed above. Before that point, identification and early assessment of disability will be likely to have at least generated a decision regarding direct financial assistance to parents in the form of Child Disability Allowance, the most common basic service provided for families in the early years, along with the generic services provided to all children who have care and protection issues. These latter services, the responsibility of the Ministry of Child, Youth and Family, do include some element of family support for care of children with intellectual disabilities, e.g. respite/long-term placement costs, but these are generally swamped by the 'protection' element of the ministry's remit. My discussions with the two parents' groups and others suggested that funding for 'respite' was only usually available if the Ministry of Health Disability Support Services would fund it, after assessment through the NASC process and referral to a Family Group conference. This also applies for more extensive 'out of family care', i.e. situations where the child is more or less permanently placed with an agency.

As in all the countries, developments in both general child care practice and specifically in disability thinking on inclusion have meant that the great majority of children are brought up in the family home, and the agencies and support groups I spoke to are geared to this aim. Objective 13 of the NZDS, which seeks to 'Enable disabled children and youth to lead full and active lives' (Minister for Disability Issues 2001) emphasizes, in its following 'Actions', 'the participation and inclusion' of disabled children in generic services for all children, and while it does not mention the notion of maintenance in families as an objective or an action, it is implicit in, for example, Action 13.5, which will look to 'Provide access for disabled children, youth *and their families*, to child, youth *and family focused* support, education, health care services, rehabilitation services, recreation opportunities and training.' At the pre-school level, this seems to have resulted in a degree of inclusion in services such as playgroups, early educational advice to parents, as well as the early years child care support we have mentioned. The impression from my visits and discussions, therefore, as can be seen from the Adam's World Tour box, is that New Zealand is similar to the Scandinavian countries in respect of services regarding birth and early childhood, albeit with the beginnings of the effect of the service marketplace, but in a minor way.

ADAM'S WORLD TOUR

Conceived in New Zealand – what next?

If Adam were now conceived in New Zealand, he would still have a good chance of being born, but the chances appear to be more affected in by where exactly his parents were living, especially the difference between urban and rural areas. In the cities, especially Auckland, there appears to be pressure for screening more mothers than just the over-35s, who are almost routinely tested, though still largely via amniocentesis for Down's syndrome, currently under review. Assuming Adam was born, we would probably be given advice about support from a local voluntary and/or parentally organized agency, usually via the early visitors from our local health service. As a child with Down's syndrome, Adam would not be eligible for support funding under the ACC, unless there were some specific 'personal injury' regarding his birth, and even then ACC funding would only cover the results of the injury. Depending on advice, and Adam's and our reaction to his care needs, we might seek assessment via our local NASC agency for funding for such things as respite care, and we would almost certainly be advised to apply for an assessment for Child Disability Benefit. Some support might also be available for assistance at pre-school educational services, depending on how this was allocated to our local area. If we were not very good at 'pushing' for things for Adam, getting information about what was available would depend on whether local support groups knew about us, something which would be less likely if we were Màori or Pacific Island people, though there would be a higher chance of family/ whànau support within those two cultures. If we were in touch with advice agencies, then preparation of applications, etc. for Adam's inclusion in the education system would also be more likely to be forthcoming – if not, Adam might even reach compulsory school age before support from the service system was offered, though the New Zealand Disability Strategy tries its best to avoid this situation.

Rowing gently down the mainstream – ORRS, educational services, and inclusion

The young man whose story opened this chapter was in the process of going through the mainstream school system. In discussion with those involved with him, it became clear that his story, while by no means unique, was not as common as Objective 3 of the NZDS would wish it to be. Objective 3 and its Actions are one of the clearest indicators, to this observer, of the influence of both normalization/SRV and the social model on the NZDS, with its powerful, ambitious, if hard to measure, statement to 'Provide the best education for disabled people' (Minister for Disability Issues 2001). The 'Actions' certainly reveal that the New Zealand government considers the 'best' education to be an inclusive one, with many references to training, communication, equitable access to resources, and other measures to 'Ensure that no child is denied access to their local, regular school because of their impairment' (ibid.: 20).

In discussion with both parents and teachers, two earlier changes in educational practice and governance came across as having affected the system's ability to meet the ambitions of the NZDS. One had to do with reforms in the governance of *all* schools, based on a report called *Tomorrow's Schools* (DoE 1988), which set up three independent Crown Entities (including a Special Education Service which advised the then predominantly separate Special

Schools). More importantly, locally elected, individual school governing bodies (Boards of Trustees) were created.

That situation has continued to the present, but was then followed by further change in the governance and funding of 'special education'. Begun in 1996, but known as Special Education 2000 (SE2000), and following at least in part the inclusive education path, these reforms sought to bring special education much more into mainstream provision. A follow-up review (Barwick 2002) resulted, among other things, in the eventual amalgamation of the SES within the Ministry of Education, and fed into the inclusive educational aspects of the NZDS. An added issue is raised with the education of Màori children, including those with intellectual disabilities. In a pilot study conducted by Poutama Pounamu, and run in parallel with a similar study on *pàkehà* schools led by Patricia O'Brien, under the overall heading of 'Enhancing Effective Practice in Special Education' (DoE 2003), the additional point in relation to the issue of individual choice is summed up for me by the following statement from their findings:

> From a Māori worldview there are no individual benefits but rather collective ones, where interdependence is just as valid as independence. These collective benefits provided a platform for generating effective practices that enhanced and sustained the cultural, social and learning needs of all who participated.
>
> (DoE 2004)

This is not to over-romanticize Màori culture as naturally conducive to inclusive education – indeed there are issues of hierarchy and gender that would certainly exercise some inclusive education proponents, but merely to point out that the cultural values of relationships and genealogy at least bear on the tendency in the *pàkehà* community for individual competition and 'choice' to dictate developments in education, often to the detriment of children with intellectual disabilities (O'Brien, P. 2005).

Going back to the inclusion issue in general, however, we need to note the effect of finance attached to specific individuals, which came in two forms, known together as the Ongoing and Renewable Resourcing Scheme (ORRS). All schools receive a grant called the Special Education Grant (SEG), and most have access to school-based resource teachers, but support beyond what those resources can cover which is the concern of ORRS. Application for ORRS funding is carried out in the same way for both schemes, the Renewable and the Ongoing. The difference, assuming the child is deemed to have needs which meet the basic criteria, is the assessment of whether the support will be needed throughout school life (Ongoing) or may change. In the latter case, the support is time-limited (Renewable). Criteria for ORRS are determined centrally, and applied by independent verifiers who work under the management control of the Ministry of Education. The key factor appears to be the definition of 'severity' of difficulty – with learning, hearing, vision, mobility, language use and social communication. 'Extreme or severe' difficulty with any of those, or 'moderate to high' difficulty combining learning and two of the others, is sufficient for some level of ORRS funding (DoE 2006) with further division of successful applicants into two differently funded levels of 'High' or 'Very High' needs. Parents normally need to approach an 'appropriate person' to complete the standard application form, decisions on which are made by three people (who review the form independently, then consolidate their view) who have never met their child, and this was the crux of concerns raised in conversations with parents. Looking at the above criteria, I am not sure where I would have put Adam at the age of 5, let alone someone who had never met him.

An increase was noted, by people I talked to, in physical resources to those schools who choose to major in special education, including some set up specifically as 'special schools', and also the growth of the population of children defined as being on the 'autistic spectrum' with their concomitant very specific demands in terms of schooling. To parents of such children, as well as those with physical as well as intellectual impairments, these 'new' or 'specialist' schools can come as a vision of relief from the fighting for such resources in the mainstream school. It is therefore not surprising that the overall impression of the school situation for children with intellectual disabilities is one of considerable variation, maintaining the (possibly clashing) public policies of inclusion and choice, and being subject in practice to the local decisions of school principals and trustees, and national decisions on the capping of the ORRS and other special education budgets. That being said, stories such as that of the young man at the beginning of this chapter appeared to be far from rare.

We have dwelt at length on the issue of funding, and of course this is far from the whole story regarding how inclusive an education a child receives. Teachers trained in the heady days of the late 1990s may well have imbued inclusion as their key value base, an important impact found by Patricia O'Brien's part of the 'Effectiveness' study cited earlier (DoE 2004). The rider to this impression, however, is that the success stories, though more numerous than many countries, do seem to depend on people, especially parents, being able to use the system, and thus, as in most market situations, to be inherently discriminatory against those with less money or political skills.

In addition, if we consider the various levels of the school system, there appear to be further differences in the applicability of inclusion. Primary schools (5–10 years), as in most countries of this study, seem to take the highest proportion of children with intellectual disabilities, diminishing, though not massively, in the intermediate (11–13) years, more so in High School/ College (14–18, or up to 21 for disabled young people). Styles of teaching, and the orientation of some secondary schools in particular to academic subjects, seem to lend themselves to both a reduction in proportions of disabled children, and the increased use of 'units' of one kind or another. In addition, the facility for disabled people, including those with intellectual disabilities, to stay on at school until 21 appears to have some deficits as well as benefits when it comes to transition to the adult world, including whether people are better served within the adult education system or remain in the school environment (O'Brien and Ryba 2005).

Looking at schooling in New Zealand compared with many of the other countries, however, it seems to this observer that the size of the population, the attempts at dealing in a sensitive and empowering way with issues for Màori and Pacific Island peoples, and the public commitment within the NZDS, have been factors in achieving a considerable amount for children with intellectual disabilities.

What this has led to for transition and adult education services is considered next, after summarizing the impression of education in New Zealand in the next Adam's World Tour box.

ADAM'S WORLD TOUR

Going to school in New Zealand

Given that we would probably have involved Adam in some sort of early childhood service, we would have been advised to work with them to apply for Adam to be assessed for ORRS funding. The fact that his intellectual disability was a 'known' one would not automatically mean he would qualify, and the form to be filled in relies on assessment of the 'degree' of his needs by the range of people who know him being accepted by assessors who do not. If we had not had much contact with early childhood services, then we might even be applying for school places without knowing about ORRS funding. The result of the ORRS application would then affect our chances of getting Adam into mainstream school, though if we chose a special school, the result of the assessment would be less important. If we did have ORRS funding, then whether it was the 'Renewable' or 'Ongoing' scheme might also affect our chances. The choice of schools is present in the NZDS, and we shouldn't be refused a place on the grounds of Adam's impairment alone, but, depending on the attitude of the principal and the trustees, some would be more welcoming than others. Even if enrolled in a mainstream school, Adam would then face a range of possibilities, from full inclusion in a regular class, through some separate lessons to a segregated 'unit' on the school campus. Adam would be more likely to be in a regular class for more of the time at primary level (up to 11) and increasingly in 'units' (or even moving to a special school) at intermediate and high school level, quite often moving to a different or substantially modified curriculum. This would also depend partly on whether his ORRS funding was moved from 'Renewable' to 'Ongoing' after the four years of the former (or whether he had ORRS funding at all). Adam could be given the opportunity to stay on at school until 21, but he would, with us, be consulted as to transition possibilities.

Out into the world, or still getting ready – transition and adult education services

In her review of the literature on transition and adult education as part of the National Advisory Committee on Health and Disability project following the NZDS, Mirfin-Veitch (2003) notes the tendency for young adults to remain in secondary schools rather than moving on to post-secondary educational settings. She also criticizes the attitude that inclusive education at this level, particularly within tertiary institutions, is seen as unimportant, or as having negative effects on the status of courses or institutions. The picture I was given on transition was that it very much depended on parents' views on (1) how much freedom of choice they sought to give to their offspring and (2) how much they were committed to an outcome involving 'real work', or regarded the issue of safe, daytime occupation as more significant. Planning for post-school in New Zealand therefore appears to fall between the stools of assumptions about the point of further education *per se* (especially if the young person has already been at school until 21) and possible routes to daytime services or employment. If it is assumed that a young person will 'never work', then they will usually be heading for 'day services' and further applications to the NASC process to fund such a move will be made. If, on the other hand, the assumption is to achieve some sort of employment, then there is an array of possibilities, funded in different ways, one of which includes the use of vocational adult education.

The transition process is thus still in development, as the Office for Disability Issues notes in its Briefing to the Incoming Minister, prepared for the 2005 General Election (ODI 2005). As for adult education, I was told of a number of courses being offered in the polytechnics in New Zealand that did address Mirfin-Veitch's comments to some extent, though again there were mixed views on their quality and availability. Where they lead will be dealt with in the next section.

Daytime services – work or occupation?

We noted, in the history section above, how workshops and other daytime activities were one of the earliest forms of service provided by IHC, and also how this demonstrated an alternative to institutional care. We also saw that, as their services and that of other agencies became the preferred alternative, hostels (later group homes) with workshops attached became commonplace (Millen 1999) and more variations on the 'workshop' theme developed. The nature of the New Zealand environment lends itself, like the farm projects in Norway, to work 'on the land' or related occupations, and many workshops or work groups carrying out this sort of work remain. With the further development of the influence of normalization/SRV and the social model, 'real work' for disabled people became more of an issue, and this certainly forms a key objective in the NZDS. Objective 4, 'Provide opportunities in employment and economic development for disabled people' has the largest number of 'Actions' – themselves divided into two sub-headings. 'Planning and training for entering employment' deals with specific vocational issues for individuals, and 'Employment and economic development', covers more macro-level policies to help the overall employment climate.

This contrasts with no *specific* reference to other daytime services within the NZDS. The emphasis on employment is echoed by the findings of, and key demands from disabled people consulted for, the *To Have an 'Ordinary' Life* document (NHC 2003). That document, however, paints a picture of daytime activities for people with intellectual disabilities much more in accord with the impression emerging from my discussions, and raises a question, noted earlier, of whether the fact that the NZDS covers all disability groups means that some of its objectives are less easily achieved for people with intellectual disabilities.

Confusion comes with the sources of funding for daytime services. A programme called 'Mainstream', run through the State Services Commission (essentially the body that covers employees of the state) seeks to assists disabled people, over a two-year period, to find work in state sector organizations. Then the Ministry of Social Development funds agencies, especially one called Workbridge, to find and oversee job finding efforts for individuals in the open market, but also funds other agencies to provide both work-type activities in sheltered workshops, and what are called 'community participation activities'. In addition, however, the Ministry of Health purchases vocational services and day activities for people who were moved out of institutions.

In most employment situations where a person's productivity is lower than the norm for the wage, employers can also apply for an Under-Rate Workers Permit, which allows payment below the minimum wage. Further still, because of the way in which finance is negotiated in terms of 'hours', in some cases, and a fixed budget in others, the amount and type of service that are funded are effectively set by NASC and the various government agencies rather than driven by need. One agency I visited, for example, was effectively being forced out of the vocational side of its business because the rates had not changed in line with costs, and thus even continuing to provide a service to existing service users was uneconomic, let alone taking on any more. Finally, the presence of a number of people with 'total packages', i.e. 24-hour care in residential homes of various sorts, distorts the picture of those seeking work, since for many people receiving such care, daytime activities come as part of the package, and often mean simply spending the day in the residence or going about with the resident group. Concerns regarding people with intellectual disabilities are therefore still being expressed in line with the findings of *To Have an 'Ordinary' Life*:

> Very few adults with an intellectual disability are in paid work. Those who are may need some ongoing support in the workplace or in seeking a new job. Many adults work in sheltered workshops or segregated work teams, where they are generally paid a minimal amount . . . with some notable exceptions, many vocational and day services do not have a developmental or future-focused approach . . . support for education, recreation and leisure tends to focus on repetitive activities designed for a group, rather than focusing on individual's goals and development . . . many adults with an intellectual disability and their families or *whànau* expressed . . . frustration at what they described as 'life-wasting' activities . . . They did not want to continue to be part of services that were segregated, custodial and meaningless . . . The poor fit of these services was particularly evident for younger adults with an intellectual disability. Many . . . had been through mainstream schooling but found when they left school that there were very few options available to them.

(NHC 2003: 34)

It is ironic that what could be called 'success' for the radical thinkers of the 1980s and 1990s, first in increasing inclusion in school, then in the whole sweep of the NZDS, should have increased expectation, and therefore frustration, at the difficulty of the service system to deliver meaningful occupation and employment. Looking at the area of residential services, the challenge is perhaps more subtle, but nonetheless equally powerful.

Residential Services – 'quality housing in the community' or a 'legacy of segregation'

Both of the phrases quoted above are used within a sentence of each other in the 2005 ODI briefing, cited above. The very positive 'Actions' from Objective 8 of the NZDS, especially 8.1, to 'Increase opportunities for disabled people to live in the community with choice of affordable, quality housing' and 8.2, to 'Support disabled people living in rural areas to remain in their own communities by improving their access to services' did not seem to apply to the living situations of the great majority of adults with intellectual disabilities, apart from those living with families, that I heard about on my visit. Nor do the rest of the Actions under Objective 8, all laudable things to do with communication, access to health services and general access in terms of getting around communities, address the situation, supporting my impressions from the literature. Quotations from three studies summarize the picture.

> More than 6,000 adults with an intellectual disability (around half of those requiring regular support) live in 'residential care' . . . They have little choice about where they live, the people they live with, and what happens in their home. Their personal freedoms are often restricted . . . no choice about what to eat, no privacy, no key to the door, and little, or no, say about being moved from one house to another . . . The historical practice of collective living, which in the past occurred in large institutions, has been transposed to what is now called community living.
>
> (NHC 2003: 22)

> It appears that services in New Zealand and elsewhere remain largely focused on the traditional model of facility funding and group homes.
>
> (MacArthur 2003: 69)

> The current collective and custodial model of service delivery must be seriously challenged. It is not possible for New Zealand Disability Strategy objectives . . . to be achieved while this single model approach to supporting the lives of people dominates.
>
> (access ability 2003: 29)

The power of the 'single model', despite some small experiments in individualized funding (ODI 2005) is compounded by virtue of these very buildings being perceived as the radical alternative to the institutions that organizations such as IHC developed. Though, as MacArthur (2003: 60) and many others who have reviewed the literature internationally, conclude, there is, in terms of what is regarded as 'best practice', agreement on 'the need for more individualised, person-centred approaches to planning and providing support in the community' and on the desirability of 'a move away from programme or facility-based models which simply reinvent institutional living in the community', the reality is somewhat different. Interpretations of what is meant by 'individualised, person-centred approaches'; the powerful interests of agencies in terms of their investment of capital resources, especially if these are originally parent-led agencies such as IHC; the greater ease with which 'programme or facility-based models' can deal with the funding processes; and indeed the views of many parents, all combine to provide a powerful force in maintaining the status quo. The other factor is the competitive market in services in New Zealand, with many agencies offering advice to parents also having a vested interest in those families being clients of the agency. Getting funding thus becomes the key issue, especially in residential services, rather than what you are getting funding for. It is interesting that a UK organization advocating segregated 'village' communities, Rescare, which gained considerable influence in the 1990s in the home country (Cox and Pearson 1995) should have now found a voice in New Zealand (Rescare NZ 2007) and that segregated 'gated villages' are not only being considered, but one has actually been put in place near Tauranga, despite the NZDS. In addition, the fact that the project to close one of the remaining large institutions, on the North Island, is managed through a joint venture by the Ministry of Health and the so-called 'Community *Group* Housing' (my emphasis), part of the 'Housing New Zealand Corporation' rather than the latter agency's regular housing provision, provides further weight to the perception that, not only is the group home as the default option still very much to the fore, but that other, even more institutional, services have come back on to the radar. Such ventures also, of course, make it easier for the agencies running such homes to claim that they actually represent the 'quality housing in the community' spoken of in Objective 8 of the NZDS.

'Non-direct' services – more important in the marketplace?

New Zealand, more than any of the other countries in this book, illustrates the tensions inherent in different cultural views of both the roles, and the rights, of the two parties involved in the life of an intellectually disabled person, the person themselves and their family. The NZDS and the actual practice of services raise the contrast between the increasing individualism and break-up of extended families and the extended 'caring' perceived to be (and in many cases actually) needed by families for their disabled member (Ballard 1994; Mirfin-Veitch et al. 2003). Beyond this, however, the acknowledgement in the NZDS of the need for a distinct set of issues regarding Màori and Pacific Island disabled people has, as a key element, different cultural views on the role of family. The very need to use the phrase 'family/*whànau*' in writing about these issues illustrates the point.

Support for 'responsibilities over and above those faced by other families' (ODI 2005: 45) is, as we have seen in this chapter, a matter of accessing services, battles over access and funding criteria, finding information, and, above all, struggling to have a voice in the future of one's offspring. Financial benefits to people as they become adults add to the dilemma. The irony of the situation is that the parental voice can be, at one and the same time, more influential than is the case for non-disabled children as they move into adulthood but also more helpless in the face of the pressures of budgets and service assessment criteria and demands, in tension with the financial pressures of benefits, that the son or daughter is given 'choice' in their lives. The lack of automatic entitlement, and the situation of what is offered by way of services, especially, as we have seen, residential services, mean the efforts of families in New Zealand seem to be taken up as much with *securing* services as using them. There is also, on the issue of 'leisure services' a corollary to the large majority of adults with intellectual disabilities being in the family home, which is the assumption that the family will then also take care of 'fun' for people. So people become either reliant on group activities if they are in residential care, or on doing things with their parents if they are living at home (NHC 2003). It is almost as if, having to fight so hard for access to the basic services in daytime and residential care, there is an assumption that leisure is a luxury that cannot be afforded, or should still be looked after by parents.

Further issues are then raised when it comes to the account that needs to be taken of the cultural issues, especially of parents, of Màori and Pacific peoples. It is interesting that the sections on this issue in the 2005 ODI briefing immediately precede an acknowledgement of the need for greater support for families. It would be presumptuous of me, as a foreign *pàkehà*, to comment on the cultural norms of either of those groups, and I did not spend time with Màori groups, and only briefly with the Pacific Island mother discussed above. There is, however, at least attention being paid to these groups in New Zealand, involving acknowledgement of the historical disadvantage that both Màori and Pacific Island groups of people have suffered, the legacy of which comes in many socio-economic indicators, but, more importantly in my view, expresses a need to develop culturally appropriate disability support services. These have come into effect, but in a limited way, and generally appear to be only for Màori. There also appear to be some issues regarding what the ODI describe as 'appropriate disability support services' for the Màori culture and the fact that, in their view, 'mainstream support services tend not to be appropriate for Pacific peoples'. The government seems to be caught in something of a three-way bind between aspects of Màori and Pacific Island peoples' culture, especially to do with roles within the family and wider *whànau*, the liberal assumptions behind both normalization/SRV and the social model, and the reality of facility and programme based services (O'Brien, P. 2005).

The role of parents and families then leads to a complementary issue, namely the apparently limited amount of *independent* advocacy services in New Zealand. Many agencies exist to give advice to, and campaign on behalf of, parents of people with intellectual disabilities, but most are either parts of bigger organizations, such as IHC or CCS, or small, local groups of parents and professionals. The young man noted at the start of this chapter had a group of people involved in his life, along the model of 'Circles of Friends' (Falvey et al.

1997), and there are other such initiatives for individuals, but I was only aware of one independent programme along the line of what might be called 'citizen advocacy'. We saw in the Scandinavian countries that the power of FUB and NFU to advocate for people with intellectual disabilities was assisted strongly by their *not* being involved in service provision. What we also saw, however, was relatively less in terms of self-advocacy, and certainly the balance of emphasis placed on self-advocacy in New Zealand and the other countries of this book was not apparent in Scandinavia. Action 2.6 in Objective 2 of the NZDS calls on government to 'Investigate the level of access that disabled people have to independent advocacy, and address any shortfall in service provision' and though the Briefing to the Minister of 2005 has clearly investigated and found a number of 'not-for-profit disability organisations' providing various forms of support, including advocacy, the 'shortfall' appears, in the ODI's view, to be in the lack, within those organizations, of the 'skills, knowledge and capacity to play a full and effective role' (ODI 2005: 23). This accords with the level of such advocacy I came across and was told about on my visit, including, in an incident I witnessed but am unable to give details of, the degree to which funding for 'independent' advocacy seemed to have certain strings attached, if its efforts involved a perception of criticism of government agencies.

ADAM'S WORLD TOUR

An adult citizen of New Zealand

By the time Adam reached the age of 18, if we as parents were active and aware of the system, we would have been in touch with a number of agencies for advice about the future of what he might be doing towards getting a job and possibly leaving home. If he had been fully included in a mainstream school, the daytime part of such planning might have also been addressed in some sort of transition plan involving, possibly, courses at a polytechnic of a vocational nature and/or work experience. If he was at a special school, or strongly segregated 'unit' in a mainstream school, such planning might well have taken place, but would be more likely to have steered Adam towards some form of sheltered workshop or other daytime 'community participation', as well as it being more likely that he would stay on at school until he was 21. If we were Màori, then Adam may well have gone to a Màori school, and then into Màori-run services, though again this would depend a lot on the efforts of parents and *whànau* and where we were in the country. If we were from the Pacific culture, less specific schooling would have been possible, and we may have kept Adam within the family support system, with little change as he grew to adulthood, unless we as parents made efforts to deal with the pākehā service system, a difficult exercise, especially in terms of awareness on both sides.

The transition to work might have led Adam to the possibility of open employment, but so might an application via Workbridge to one of the job-finding agencies, or for funding through the Mainstream scheme for a job with a government agency. This seems to apply more to people with physical impairments, however, though there is seasonal work in the rural areas that also includes people with intellectual disabilities.

If we, and/or Adam, wanted him to move away from home, then it would again depend on our resourcefulness, contacts and support. If we got the support of an agency committed to an individual solution for Adam, they would help us with a proposal to the NASC system (who may well have known of us anyway) for approval for funding. The sort of solution would depend a lot on the attitude of the agency, and a limited number would be able to propose solutions that fitted in with Adam's and our wishes. The majority, however, would be more constrained in what could be offered, with a place in a group home of 4–6 or more people being the most common, depending also on the rurality of the area in which we lived. If Adam were someone with more severe impairments than he has as a person with Down's syndrome, then he might be part of experimental schemes in totally individualized funding. More likely Adam would remain living in the family home, especially if we did not push for change in the situation.

As the final Adam's World Tour box implies, therefore, services in New Zealand seem to require greater efforts than in Scandinavia for parents of people with intellectual disabilities to achieve 'an ordinary life' with and for their offspring. The range of funding sources and access points, the effective rationing of services and the variety of service agencies in the welfare market all put a heavy burden of persistence, commitment, political awareness and articulacy on parents, with the additional twist of the cultural history of New Zealand. What would be seen, given the theoretical roots of the NZDS in normalization/SRV and the social model, as the 'success' of getting a national publicly expressed policy so close to those roots and, as this is written, one which has enabled New Zealand to lead, and get assent to, a new United Nations Convention on Rights of Disabled People (ODI, 2006), has to be tempered by the ability of the model of service finance and governance to deliver that policy.

5 Australia

Who pays; who cares?

The Walrus and the Carpenter
Were walking close at hand;
They wept like anything to see
Such quantities of sand:
'If this were only cleared away',
They said, 'it would be grand!'

'If seven maids with seven mops
Swept it for half a year,
Do you suppose', the Walrus said,
'That they could get it clear?'
'I doubt it', said the Carpenter.
And shed a bitter tear.

(Lewis Carroll)

INSTANT IMPACTS

Australia – meaningful days?

Two young men with Down's syndrome illustrate a significant issue in Australian services. Arrangements for funding mean 'employment' services are largely funded by the federal government (hereafter 'Commonwealth') whereas 'residential services' and, more relevant here, 'community-based activities' are funded by the individual States and Territories (hereafter STs), sometimes on a shared basis with the Commonwealth. Within these definitions, however, 'employment' does not only mean open employment, but also attendance at places that could be called 'segregated settings' that carry out 'business services'. The financing regimes can therefore produce some anomalies in terms of how very similar people, such as the two young men, both in their thirties and with similar ability levels, are 'classed'. One worked in what was very obviously, in terms of the setting, the type of work, and the payment to workers, what an outside observer would call 'real work', though essentially a 'sheltered workshop'. I met the young man who worked there in the scheduled coffee break for all workers, kept to time by the factory hooter, and he told me of his work making 'day-glo' jackets for people in jobs where they need to be readily seen. We did not have much time to talk about the rest of his life, as the hooter went and he had to return to work. There was still less conversation with the young man in the other location, however, despite the fact that he was sitting doing not very much, in the room of the day centre where he and eight other people were undertaking 'community activities' by listening to music from a 'ghetto-blaster'. The young man and one other person in the group were physically able, and could talk, whereas the others had varying, but significant, degrees of physical and mental impairment, and very limited speech. I was taken into the room, and given details of the people therein, but not encouraged to talk to them.

Two men, in two different places in the daytime, not because of their level of need, still less their individual preference, but because of the funding granted to each by the different systems. As we shall see, this was a big issue across the country, with some people getting no funding at all after leaving school, some getting 'transition' money, which then ends after a couple of years, and others offered places in whichever of the agencies receiving money from the two funding streams has vacancies. It also illustrates that matters of funding do not just differ between countries, but also within countries, and that the benefits of so-called 'individualized funding' are not without their drawbacks.

Introduction

On my first, and only other, visit to Australia and New Zealand in 1997, attending and presenting on a series of workshops given by Wolf Wolfensberger and his associates, the great majority of my time was spent in lecture halls and discussions on the issues of the workshops. There was little time, therefore, to get to know the culture of the two countries. Despite this, the earlier visit still highlighted the much greater Màori presence in New Zealand, as compared with the aboriginal people of Australia. This was reinforced much more powerfully on the latest visit, when I was much more aware of the limited presence, even in 2005, of the indigenous peoples of Australia in political affairs, in national and state governments, and simply in terms of a physical presence in the urban centres that make up the majority of the living places of that country. Though some progress has been made since his remarks, the views, in 1995, of Terry O'Shane, a Commissioner with the Australian and Torres Strait Islander Commission, chime strongly with my impressions:

Australia was settled by the British, using the doctrine of *Terra Nullius* as a legal entitlement to claim ownership of the entire land . . . At that moment Australia witnessed a so-called civilized people denying the indigenous peoples of this country any rights as a peoples (*sic*) . . . *Terra Nullius* meant that we, indigenous people, were not a people. We were a life form without intellect . . .

We were a people who have a history in Australia of between 50–100,000 years . . . We understood profoundly the intricate workings of nature, with a comprehensive knowledge of the seasons . . . we had unmatched survival skills but were treated as though we, as a people, had intellectual disabilities.

(quoted in O'Brien and Murray 1997: 61)

Having recognized that common oppression, there will, as already noted, be little more on indigenous people in this chapter. The overwhelming nature of their separateness and lower social status, even today, as reflected in a myriad of statistics of poverty, relative criminal convictions, deaths in custody, and illiteracy, despite land claim cases and other gradual symbols of recognition, means that intellectual disability is lost as a specific issue (Peterson and Sanders 1998). Feeling guilty about colluding, in effect, with this marginalization of indigenous peoples, I nevertheless have to leave the matter there, if I am going to present an honest impression of the situation in Australian services.

Ironically, perhaps, the other key difference from New Zealand, namely the different powers and responsibilities of STs and the Commonwealth will be dealt with at length. As we shall see, that difference is a key part of some major problems that seem to be besetting the lives of people with intellectual disabilities and their families. Before that, however, the summary of the history of services below raises some familiar themes.

Historical development of services

Colonies in the colonies – early institutions

Two quotations sum up, for me, the history of services in Australia up to the major changes in the 1980s and 1990s which form the basis of current arrangements. The first is a moving reminder that the roots of the history of intellectual disability go deep. Written by a lawyer involved with a coroner's inquiry into the deaths of nine men at a Melbourne institution in 1996, Ian Freckleton's words still cast a chill through many of us immersed in the niceties of academic argument about theories of disability:

On a bleak day in October 1996 a strange procession wended its way through Kew Residential Services ('Kew Cottages'). At the time Kew

Cottages accommodated approximately 600 residents with intellectual disabilities, aged between 21 and 68 years, and contained 28
residential units or wards . . . said by those who ran the institution to
be designed, as far as possible, to provide a home-like atmosphere. Kew
Cottages was originally built in the grounds of Willsmere Hospital in
1887 . . . situated on about 40 hectares of parkland on a picturesque
hill overlooking the sprawling expanse of Melbourne. By 1996 it had
experienced a series of changes and expansions, making it one of the
larger remaining 'total institutions' in Victoria . . . It was a modest
walk to Building 37 where, six months before, nine men with intellectual disabilities had perished in a fire . . . The unit was a serpentine
construction with multiple rooms. It had housed 46 men before the
conflagration . . . We walked up the melange of Victorian buildings
and post-war prefabricated structures that were home for so many
people whom the community never has the opportunity to see.
Strange noises that the carers could not quell erupted from some of
the buildings as we passed . . .

The men who died . . . were hardly ever named during the inquest
. . . somewhat symbolic of how their lives had been lived. They were
aged between 31 and 61 . . . and most had lived at Kew Cottages for
many years . . . It was possible to see where their beds had been and
that a number of the men had crumpled to the floor and, presumably,
died of asphyxiation without being able to leave their rooms or escape
through the labyrinthine construction to safety.

(Freckleton 2005: 77–8)

Errol Cocks's address to the Chief Executives of ACROD (the National Industry
Association for Disability Services) not only confirms the message of the opening quotation, but wryly brings us to the present day:

It is interesting to reflect briefly on what a meeting like this one would
have looked like in the disability sector right up to the middle of the
20th century. Rather than a meeting of CEOs or professional managers, this would be a meeting of superintendents of large institutions, probably mainly consisting of psychiatrists or at least medically
qualified *men*. Like this conference, there would be many topics
on how best to manage disability, however, the purpose would be
expressed quite differently. The superintendents would have taken
pride in their role to protect society from the people they cared for in
their institutions and to provide asylum, with limited attention given
to the quality of the care being provided, at least from a modern
perspective.

(Cocks 2005: 1)

In his penetrating and provocative book, *Lives Unrealised* (2003), Rob Westcott not only gives a significant analysis of the situation of learning disabilities in the industrialized world, but also a detailed analysis of the history of services in his native Australia. He includes Kew Cottages in his list of early Australian institutions, citing it as one of the first to pay any attention to education and training of inmates. The asylums had contained both people with intellectual disabilities and mental illness, and, as elsewhere, separation of those groups did not fully occur for many years. For a brief period, Kew became known as the site of the first large-scale attempt at a curative and education programme geared exclusively to 'idiots and imbeciles' anywhere in Australia, with 60 children placed in the first three cottages. Like the other countries that we have already discussed, optimism about education, rare as it was in Australia, was quickly swallowed up by the demands for incarceration and segregation of the eugenics movement at the turn of the century. Thus not just children, but adults, were taken in to the ever-expanding institution, and, noting (ibid.: 115) that the mortality rate in 1950, at 20 per cent, was at an all-time high, comparing *un*favourably with the 7 per cent of Kew's opening years, Westcott goes on to sum up its history in typically forthright fashion:

> Kew Cottages is not at all unique. The same sorry spectacle of human neglect was played out throughout Australia in the first half of the Twentieth Century. Children with mild intellectual disabilities frequently remained at home with struggling families. As adults they often continued to be dealt with by the judicial system, regardless of whether they had committed any crime. Those with more significant disabilities usually found their way to the institutions established grudgingly by governments which self applauded their humanitarianism and remained blind to the truth: that people with disabilities were dying or living in endless suffering in Australia's institutions years after the genocide of their peers in Germany had been halted.
>
> (Westcott 2003: 117)

As we have seen in all the earlier chapters, few countries were without their eugenic policies. Australia also had distinct views on other groups who might be thought of as 'unfit'. Writing in 1911, a Doctor Birmingham of the Western Australian Lunacy Department put it clearly enough:

> The evil arising from the unchecked increase in defectives is growing and spreading throughout the civilized world, forcing its way into all classes of society and vitiating the health of the nation. We are careful that no black skins lie found in our white Australia, but we are doing

nothing to protect the transmission of degenerate brains to those who come after us.

(Birmingham 1911, quoted in Cocks et al. 1996: 66)

Eugenics Down Under

So with a 'white Australia' twist, STs began to put into practice similar measures to other countries. The Eugenics Society of New South Wales was founded in 1912, segregative legislation was passed in South Australia in 1913 and Tasmania in 1920, and various ST parliaments debated sterilization bills in the 1930s. Though the war and, possibly, some inkling of what had happened in Germany meant that these never became law, eugenic views, societies and debates continued, as did, of course the segregation of people with intellectual disabilities. On the education scene, already excluding children with intellectual disabilities, the great expansion of state education also retained the strong influence of eugenics. As one educationalist puts it, the news was good for a while:

> Grading and sorting survived the Second World War, albeit in revised forms, cleansed by amnesia of its eugenics lineage, and formed the growth of larger and larger 'factory schools' into the 70's and 80's, where, at the societal level in Australia, we had the highest employment and lowest unemployment rates in the Western world. This was indeed our golden era.
>
> (Wills 2005: 57)

But then comes the sting in the tail (ibid.):

> People with disability labels were never a part of the 'good life era' for their sorting occurred before grade one. The old IQ made sure of that . . . The fact that we originally 'sorted and segregated' for eugenic purposes was forgotten and in its place we began to think segregation served a pedagogical purpose.

Post-war changes – parents and normalization

So the familiar pattern of eugenics, institutions, and segregation continued in Australia after the war. The impact of normalization was felt, to a limited extent, in the 1970s, with the publication of the *New Patterns* and *Normalization* books, visits by Nirje and others to Australia and visits to Nebraska and Ontario by a number of young and influential individuals (Millier 1999). In terms of actual effects, however, change was initially more about, in the ironic phrase used by Freckleton above, making the institutions more 'homelike'. Most were still run by the Commonwealth government, as part of the Psychiatric Health department, though the normalization influence, together with pressure from parents and the growth of some charitable agencies with a more developmental focus (Chenoweth 2000) seems to have been influential in changing things in some STs. Queensland, for example, decided in the late 1960s to separate intellectual disability from the psychiatric hospital system, resulting in the development between the Health Department, Children's Services and the Kelvin Grove College of Advanced Education, of a three-year Associate Diploma in Residential Care, and, by 1977 a new branch (Intellectual Handicap Services) of the Psychiatric Services Division of the Health Department. I met someone who claimed to have been in the 'last cohort' of 'mental handicap nurses' and qualified in 1977. As in other countries, parents in Australia got together regarding services, and found a ready set of ideas in normalization and then its development into SRV. Because of the greater powers of STs over services, however, this did not materialize into a *national* campaigning or service-providing organization, such as IHC in New Zealand, but seems to have been more about particular leaders and different negotiations and alliances with ST bureaucrats sympathetic to their views (Mackay 2006). There were national gatherings of parents groups, still present in the National Council on Intellectual Disability, and the national Down Syndrome Association, and there were some large-scale services set up at ST level, or even straying over borders, but since STs controlled the finances, issues at that level were more distinct. In this regard, it is interesting that Queensland, as we shall see, seems to be one of the strongest STs for small parent-led services and campaigning groups of parents, but also contains very large organizations stemming from parent-led roots. Following the 1977 reorganization noted above, Queensland began moving people out of the 'Training Centres' (the institutions) into the community, into 'group homes', normally with six people sharing. This contrasts, to some degree, with the growth of 'hostels', 15–25 bedded dwellings in community settings, as the alternative to hospitals in other STs.

The bureaucratic influence is also mentioned by Millier (1999), when he reflects on the effect of a 1980 visit by Wolfensberger on State and Commonwealth policymakers, referring to COMSERV, a planning system for services with which Wolfensberger had been heavily involved during his time at NIMR in Toronto (NIMR 1974; Race 2003). This formed part of a workshop he gave on Planning Comprehensive Service Systems, and Millier notes its influence on *New Directions* (Handicapped Programs Review (Australia) 1985), established by the Commonwealth government in 1983, pointing out that, whatever the dislike of 'all things American' and the academic vitriol thrown about in the 1980s as the social model of disability also had its effects, both *New Directions* and the subsequent national 1986 Disability Services Act contain language inescapably tied up with normalization/SRV.

Chenoweth (2000) concurs with Millier, and notes the effect on both policy development and training as the STs moved to formulate their own responses to the Disability Services Act of 1986 and then the Disability Discrimination Act of 1992. Many people from the SRV network I spoke to on my visit described this period, roughly the decade from 1987–97, as SRV's 'golden era' with the specific Wolfensberger SRV formulation becoming adopted by the radical 'movement' following the first full SRV and PASSING workshop given by Michael Kendrick in 1987. That period also saw the firming up of the national Australian SRV Group (ASG) which continues to the present, though again the greater ST orientation of services has meant that SRV initiatives have been pursued more powerfully by local groups such as Values in Action in Queensland.

The sorts of values statements contained in the first, 1991, and subsequent two versions of the Commonwealth States and Territories Disability Agreement (CSTDA) (Office of Disability 1991, 1997, 2003) clearly reflect the influence of SRV, and the 1990s saw the greatest number of visits and consultancies by the international SRV networks, culminating in an extensive series of workshops by Wolfensberger and his colleagues in 1997.

The ST/Commonwealth situation continues to be a sore point, however, and of course, as we shall see in the detailed descriptions of services below, the CSTDA has remained in force. Other events beyond SRV or intellectual disability, in particular the neo-conservative agenda of the Howard government in the new millennium and the Australian version of managerialism, have also had their effect, however, all contributing to the service system whose details form the rest of this chapter.

Services in Australia – an impression

In its annual publication of statistics on usage of the CSTDA, the government quotes from the 'preamble to the Agreement'. The influences, as noted above, of SRV and other sources are clear:

> The Agreement is based on '*the premise that communities are enriched by the inclusion of people with disabilities and that positive assumptions about the gifts and capacities of people with disabilities, including those with high support needs, are fundamental to their experience of a good life and to the development and delivery of policy, programs and services*'.
>
> The Agreement '*recognises that both levels of government fulfil complementary roles in the development and delivery of public policy and services, and that both have a pivotal role in promoting the rights, equality of opportunity, citizenship and dignity of people with disabilities*'.
>
> (Australian Healthcare Associates 2005; italics in original)

The Introduction goes on (ibid.: 6), in a section headed 'Building on Previous Agreements' to note the periods (1991–1996, 1997–2002) of the previous two agreements, and, in a telling phrase, to note that the current Agreement 'reflects the current policy environment and the significant reforms and initiatives on which all governments have embarked'. This phrase should be noted as we proceed to the detail below, but first the usual overview is provided in Table 5.1. As noted, and put simply, the Commonwealth deals with Employment services

Table 5.1 Schematic overview of 'services' that affect the lives of people with intellectual disabilities in Australia

'Service'	Formal organizational place	Specialist or generic?	Main source(s) of funding
Pre-natal services	ST hospitals and health centres Medical practices Private hospitals and practitioners	Generic and specialist	ST Health departments Health Insurance
Post-natal and early childhood services	ST hospitals and health centres Medical practices Private hospitals and practitioners Early childhood agencies, some voluntary	Generic clinical services, but agency input varying in specialization	ST Health departments Health Insurance ST funding under CSTDA headings 'Community support services' HACC funding – joint State/ Territory & Commonwealth
Non-educational services for children	Agencies, including those providing respite services	Specialist and generic	ST funding under CSTDA headings 'Community support services' HACC funding
Education services – children and young adults	Local School Boards Independent school trusts	Generic and specialist	ST Education department funding to Local School Boards for 'government schools' – Commonwealth funding for 'non-government' schools
Education services – adults	TAFE	Generic and specialist	General ST tertiary education funding
Residential services – adults	Agencies – some ST direct provision Some public housing	Generic and specialist	ST funding under CSTDA headings 'Accommodation' or 'Respite' – HACC funding for in home respite

(Continued overleaf)

Table 5.1 Continued

'Service'	Formal organizational place	Specialist or generic?	Main source(s) of funding
Daytime services – non-work	Agencies	Largely specialist	ST funding under CSTDA headings 'Community support services' and 'Community Access services'
Daytime services – work	Agencies, either supported employment or 'business services	Largely specialist	Commonwealth funding under CSTDA heading 'Employment services' – administered through 'case-based funding' from July 2006
Leisure assistance	Agencies – usually as part of broader package	Largely specialist	ST funding under CSTDA heading 'Community Access services'
Advocacy services	Agencies, including parent support agencies, individual Citizen advocacy agencies, and campaigning organizations	Specialist	Commonwealth and ST funding under CSTDA heading 'Advocacy, information and print disability services'
Financial Assistance	Commonwealth agency 'Centrelink'	Specialist within generic service	Commonwealth general social security funding
Parental 'support services'	Acting as all parents Also setting up individual or community agency	Specialist, in that all children are different	Own finances, or individual funding for various aspects of CSTDA

and Advocacy, with the STs covering the rest, sharing Advocacy with the Commonwealth. Note that the CSTDA does not cover education at school.

What, then, does this mean for a child born, or in fact conceived in Australia in 2005 in terms of the impact of those services on their lives? As usual, we start before birth.

Pre-natal services – moving which way?

A couple of weeks before I arrived in Canberra, the press reported that the High Court had been asked to decide whether severely disabled children could sue over medical negligence which resulted in birth (Pelly 2005). What the paper described as children, although adding that one was now 24, were seeking the right to sue their mothers' doctors for 'wrongful life'. The case hinged on doctors allegedly failing to describe the consequences of the pregnancy going to term, arguing that if they had not been 'negligent' in this regard, then the 24-year-old woman (described as being 'blind, deaf, spastic and mentally retarded') would not have been born, and thus would not have had to endure 24 years of 'pain and suffering'. Similar arguments were used for a 5-year-old severely disabled boy. The report gave the impression, enhanced by subsequent conversations in different parts of Australia, that pre-natal screening was routine, and if the possibility of disability was detected, most Australian women would be encouraged to seek an abortion. What that initial impression did not reveal, however, were the differences between STs, both in the legal and policy positions. De Crespigny and Savulescu (2004: 204) put it as follows: – 'many Australian abortions, including many of those for severe fetal abnormality, occur without legal clarity'. Lawrence and Crowther (2003), surveying screening for Down's syndrome, found similar state variations, concluding that 'While providers engage in external accreditation and quality assurance programs, state and federal governments have been slow to formulate relevant policies and standards' (ibid.: 224).

The disability rights movement in Australia appears to have been less aligned on many issues with the normalization/SRV movement than seemed to be the case in New Zealand (Millier 1999; Carling-Burzacott 2004). In their critique of the oppression of certain interpretations of 'choice', however, Goggin and Newell (2005) seem to have placed the issue of abortion on the grounds of disability as a common theme between the two groups. The indication of general societal attitudes to people with intellectual disabilities provided by Australian policies on pre-natal screening and abortion is therefore perhaps not as clear as at first glance.

Early childhood services – habilitation and early intervention

As in New Zealand, early childhood first brings parents up against the intricacies of the funding system, though in Australia there is the added dimension of their particular ST's interpretation of the CSTDA. After early health-related interventions immediately following birth, parents will not automatically receive services to support them in the care of their young children. Some STs fund 'family support' type service agencies, who, while not direct providers, can give advice and support to parents and also act as 'service brokers' as their relationship with the parents develops. Other parents make their own contacts with the ST disability funding organization set up to oversee and administer the CSTDA.

Parents of young children, I was told in discussion with one of the support organizations, and confirmed by parents, are quite likely to be offered 'respite services' in the early years. This is partly because funding exists for this form of service through the Home and Community Care (HACC) funding stream as well as via the CSTDA. Respite in 'residential care' at this early stage is quite rare, partly because it is considered more desirable for such support to be given to parents in the child's own home, and partly because this would require full ST funding through the CSTDA and would be in government-provided accommodation, of which there is a limited supply. Respite in the child's own home, through HACC, which is jointly funded by the Commonwealth and the ST, is therefore more common, and the further HACC remit, to cover 'carer's needs', has the overarching aim of keeping people in family homes. In the early days, of course, many children with intellectual disabilities present not greatly different caring needs to non-disabled babies, and therefore the need for 'respite' can be less pressing than the need for support in developmental activities. On the other hand, for parents of children with multiple and/or severe disabilities, such respite can be crucial, and is often combined with specialist, often segregated medicalized pre-school units to address the needs of such children.

As children reach pre-school age, there are, in different STs, what a support agency referred to as 'bits of money' for various activities such as kindergarten places. Most parents pay for day care places for their non-disabled children, so some of this funding (plus some help from HACC if the place can be classed as 'respite') eases the financial burden on parents or enables one or both partners to remain in employment. There appeared to be a few consciously inclusive day care facilities, who are resourced to take children of all levels of ability, and more who will take children with disabilities who have 'adequate support'. ST Education Departments also fund pre-school establishments, and attendance at these can be beneficial in leading to the assessment of where the child will be offered a school place.

So, as the first Adam's World Tour box shows, there is, as would be expected from the governance and finance arrangements operating in Australia, quite a wide variation in the level and sort of services provided around the birth of a child with intellectual disabilities, but rarely is there the lack of resources that will become an issue for parents as their child grows up.

ADAM'S WORLD TOUR

Conceived in Australia – what next?

The chances of Adam being born in Australia might vary more than the impression gained from the media, or conversation with parents and others involved with services for people with intellectual disabilities. Screening would be offered if his mother were over 35, and use is being made in some STs of a test of the physical dimensions of the foetus using various scanning techniques. The legal position, however, is unclear, and the amount of testing would also vary depending on the moral position of the ST government on abortion, and the views of the medical professionals in the different maternity facilities. That would also be affected, to some extent, by whether we had insurance and used private facilities for our healthcare.

Once Adam were born, the medical supervision around birth seems to be reasonably consistent, but our use of services in Adam's early years would depend on a number of factors. First, whether we had access to support agencies that could inform us of funding possibilities, especially respite via HACC. Second, whether we were articulate and active parents, as far as establishing and using our entitlements, and third, the degree of needs generated by Adam. By the time he was coming up to school age, however, it is likely that we would be in contact with services that would assist us in preparing our case for Adam's schooling.

Education – inclusion or 'preferred school'?

Once again, we begin with the distinction between Commonwealth and ST influence and funding. A significant part of the Australian education system, like that in New Zealand, is controlled locally by School Boards, elected from the community, with representatives from various interest groups needing to be included, depending on ST interpretation of overall government policy. Unlike New Zealand, however, the financing of the two-thirds or so of schools designated as 'government schools' comes from *State and Territory* government and is controlled by ST Education Departments, who set overall strategic policies, including policies on inclusion. This still leaves a significant number, around 32 per cent (Harrington 2004) of so-called 'non-government schools'. Though STs provide supplementary assistance to non-government schools, the Commonwealth is their primary source of public funding. For government schools, the Commonwealth acts only as a supplementary funding source via particular initiatives. Most non-government schools have some religious affiliation, with approximately two-thirds of students enrolled in Catholic schools, and all have greater freedom over budgets and admission policies. This clearly has a crucial part to play when it comes to matters of inclusion, since ST policies can be circumvented, if not actually ignored. Commonwealth legislation, especially the Disability Discrimination Act of 1992 and the States Grant

(Primary and Secondary Education Assistance) Act 2000 (SGPSEA), exercises some control over both government and non-government schools, but, though individual ST policies and specific initiatives can take things further towards inclusion, they can only insist on such policies in government schools. This appears to mean that a lot depends on the Principals and Boards of individual schools, even within the government sector. When a child is approaching school age, therefore, and is likely to need support within the school system, parents will be encouraged to apply for an assessment to be carried out by people authorized by the ST Education Department. If the child meets the criteria of the SGPSEA Act, then specific national funding may be available, attached to the child.

Here we get into issues relating to legislation and policy for disability as a whole, without differentiation between different categories and levels of disabled children. Access to the Commonwealth per capita funding, however, is dependent upon funding eligibility under ST disability programmes, and thus on whether the ST interpretation of criteria defined in the SGPSEA Act, agrees with Commonwealth interpretations of those criteria.

A national government Senate Committee set up to investigate education and disabled children described the situation as follows

> the broad and untested definition of disability under the Disability Discrimination Act has been one of the stumbling blocks to final-izing education standards ... Significant increases in the number of diagnosed conditions such as Aspergers Syndrome, ADHD and learning disabilities have further increased the demand for edu-cational resources, yet there has not been a commensurate increase in Commonwealth funding to support these students.
>
> (Senate Committee Report 2002: paras 2.10–11)

The committee had earlier discussed what they considered to be the implica-tions of these definitional disputes:

> The committee recognizes that the education of students with dis-abilities is a state responsibility. The evidence suggests, however, that in supporting the education of students with disabilities, the Commonwealth has given scant regard to the obligations imposed on education authorities since the introduction of the Commonwealth's anti-discrimination legislation.
>
> (ibid.: paras 2.8–9)

Since that committee's deliberations, judging from my discussions in all three of the states I visited, the situation has not greatly developed, despite the SGPSEA Act. In the Australian Capital Territory, for example, in his

introduction to the ten-year 'vision for the ACT' produced in 2004, the Minister for Disability, Housing and Community Services still includes as 'major
challenges' which 'we will have to overcome' people's 'full access to the mainstream services in the fundamental areas of health, *education*, housing,
employment, justice and transport' (DHCS 2004: 5, my emphasis). In Queensland, too, discussions with parents and others in 2005 echoed the views of
their predecessors, when research conducted by Queensland Parents for People
with a Disability (QPPD) in 2001 on the process of decision-making around
educational choice by parents of students with disabilities found that:

- The majority of students with disability attend school at a special
  education unit or special school and do not attend the same school
  as their siblings.
- Parents said that their child would not be at the school they currently
  attend if they did not have a disability and the advice and information given to them by teachers, school officials and other professionals are often biased towards segregated education pathways and
  strongly influences the decision-making process.

(QPPD 2001)

The views of parents in all the states I visited concurred with the QPPD, and
challenge government figures as to the number of children 'included' in the
school of their parents' choice, or in mainstream classes:

Prevalence figures are very difficult to determine from one state to
another and from one system to another, for a variety of reasons.
These reasons include: systems and sectors differ in their requirements to provide information on different groups of students with
disabilities, the use of different definitions, the different ways a definition has been operationalized, the different groups for which data are
reported and the different ways on which data is collected and
reported.

(Van Kraayenoord et al. 2000: 78)

The picture, therefore was of an assessment process, which varied in detail but
not in essentials between STs, conducted by an authorized person, theoretically
in consultation with all those who know the child, and often part of a pre-
school programme. Parents are then either offered a 'preferred school', with
assistance attached, from the regular government school system, or if not a
special school – the most common seeming to be school with a 'unit', formally
identified as such or acting as such *de facto*. If parents opt for a 'non-preferred'
school, either in the non-government sector, or because they want their children with intellectual disabilities to go to the same school as their siblings and

peers, then assistance may not be offered. This can enable Principals to refuse admission on the grounds that the school cannot support the child without earmarked assistance. As in New Zealand, the overwhelming view was that persistent, mostly middle-class, parents would achieve greater success should they want a particular school that was not keen to take them, and parents of severely disabled children would be strongly pressured to take whichever offer came with funding. In both cases, the Senate Committee's finding (2002: 24) that the system encouraged 'an exaggeration of disability to secure better funding' had formed in my notes well before I came across their report.

A further common finding across the STs was the greater ease of attaining a regular school place at the primary level. When coming up to secondary level, there is a similar process of assessment, but it now appears to be harder to get into a local school if it has no unit. It also appears to be easier at primary level to have an inclusive curriculum. At secondary level (up to 14) when the academic performance of students becomes more significant, there is greater differentiation between all pupils according to their judged academic ability, and here the relatively high proportion of non-government schools in the Australian system begins to have greater significance. One of the other reasons than religious beliefs for these schools to exist is a belief that they will produce higher academic attainment generally, and the presence of children with intellectual disabilities (not necessarily other impairments) will, by definition, adversely affect a school's standing in academic league tables. The QPPD, in their response to the Senate Committee's draft report, are forthright in their view of how this affects their children's chances of attending their local school if it is in the 'private sector', wryly juxtaposing their members' experiences with the submissions from the non-government sector:

> We note the submissions from the non-government school sector are heavily weighted with financial details on the cost of supporting students with disabilities. QPPD has observed that the non-government sector uses the lack of resources to exclude students with disabilities. Yet non-government schools have greater flexibility and more choice in deciding to use their resources for this support. QPPD has gathered anecdotal evidence that even students with modest support needs are being refused enrolment. QPPD believes this is a conscious decision by the non-government sector to avoid investment in resources for students with disability. Some non-government schools actively discourage parents from enrolling by informing them that they cannot afford to support their son or daughter.
>
> (QPPD 2003)

By the time students are at the high school level (15+), the academic curriculum appears to be an even more powerful determinant of inclusion, either at all, or in a special unit. As in many countries, the vocational route for children at this level is definitely considered inferior to the academic one, and that is where you will normally find students with intellectual disabilities.

Many schools, whether or not they have a unit, will try to get work placements for their 'non-academic' students. In some STs there are schemes to assist with the transition process that specifically target such placements as a key goal, but there appears to be an uneasy relationship between schools and employment services over the relative roles of each, and there is variation in which group receives funding.

From my discussions and from the literature, and as the next Adam's World Tour box shows, it therefore seems to be the case that not a great deal of progress has been made with the Senate Committee's recommendation that:

> In the interests of reducing discrimination and promoting integration in education, the Productivity Commission considers that a general objective of government education funding arrangements should be to ensure school students with disabilities have the same range of education choices that other students have. Their choice of school sector should only be subject to the same personal factors, such as location, income and education needs as other students.
>
> (Senate Committee Report 2002: 379)

ADAM'S WORLD TOUR

Going to school in Australia

Depending on whether we had been in touch with the service system, which ST we were in, and whether we had already applied for, and been successful with, funding, Adam's pre-school programmes and entry into the school system would be very variable. Everywhere there would have been some form of assessment of Adam, carried out by the ST Education Department or individuals or agencies licensed by them, as part of an application form for individual assistance with funding. Beyond this, however, individual schools and School Boards would have their own policies, overt and covert, for admitting Adam or otherwise if we as parents wished him to go to a particular school. In most STs a 'school of choice' would have been indicated by the Education Department or their agents, and whatever individual funding we might have attracted would be geared to taking up that place. It would be more likely, if we went along with the process without much input from us as parents, that Adam would be offered a place in a mainstream school with a 'special unit' which would vary in the degree of its inclusiveness. If Adam were more severely disabled, there would be a significant chance of him being offered a place in a special school. If we wanted Adam to go to a specific school, and pushed for this, then success would depend on the attitude of the School Board and the Principal, with less likelihood of success (with arguments of 'lack of facilities') if the school were one of the approximately one-third of schools described as 'non-government schools'.

All of this would be easier to achieve at primary level, with full inclusion diminishing as Adam moved through the age range. As he reached his late teens, the possibility of transition funding (varying in quantity and form in different STs) might encourage us to try and get Adam to leave school and take up a place in 'business services' (see below). If we did not win the competition for this funding, or we thought (or were told) that Adam would be unlikely to (or 'never') work, then there would be a strong incentive to keep Adam at school as long as possible. The school would be likely to have already given Adam a work-oriented curriculum if they saw prospects of this happening, and they might also have encouraged him to move on to a TAFE (see below) - otherwise they would assist, in varying degrees, our application for funding for non-vocational services once Adam left school.

Daytime services – what is work?

A question I asked in nearly all of my meetings with parents was 'What happens when your son or daughter leaves school?' The response of a parent of a young woman with Down's syndrome, whose daughter was, in fact, in nearly full-time employment, was blunt, if dramatic – 'This is where you cut your throat!'

This lady was reflecting the wider picture, through her role with the Down Syndrome Association and other State bodies in her part of Australia, and through the national DSA. Here the working out of the CSTDA in practice comes into full play, and so discussion of the different options for activity in the daytime is less easily fitted into the categories used in earlier chapters. It is tempting, in fact, to see the provision of daytime services simply as a battleground for funding between the STs and the Commonwealth, but this would be to over-simplify the situation, and to leave aside some real ideological issues over what constitutes 'work', and how people are assessed as being 'work-ready'.

As we have seen in the first three countries, the notion of 'real work', i.e. work of a similar nature to, and paid at the same rates as, the open job market, has proved the toughest nut to crack in the provision of services to replace the all-encompassing institutions. So too, in Australia, with the added dimension, illustrated by the 'Instant Impacts' story above, of the CSDTA definition and funding of 'employment services'. Most STs have some form of 'transition' scheme, but application for funding under such schemes tends to direct a person towards the 'non-employment' route, whereas for those who envisage employment as their destination, broader Commonwealth schemes come into effect including 'business services' such as the agency attended by one of the young men in the opening story. From my discussions and reading (Brown 2003; Rollo 2005; S&S Consultants 2005; Harman 2006), it appears that when such specific 'moving on' schemes started, it was easier to get money for a 'middle group' of people, who might not be ready for work for a while, but who would benefit from meaningful daytime activities. Increasing limitations on ST budgets seem to mean that, like individual funding for education, the case now has to be made out that the individual has 'severe needs' for any funding to be forthcoming, and that it tends to come in the form of a finite number of payment 'bands', usually expressed in terms of 'hours'. Parents, sometimes in conjunction with independent advice agencies and/or providing agencies, then try to work out a 'package' from that funding. Once this has been agreed, involving the agency/ies offering a place to the person concerned, and funding arrangements being put in place with the ST disability department, then attendance begins. In one State I visited, which I was told was fairly typical nationally, the allocated sums from the State budget under the 'Community Activities' heading would buy about '11 hours' of service time at most. Parents can, of course, buy extra hours themselves, or have to do so if they do not succeed in the annual funding round, which appears as an annual lottery with many parents (Croft 2000). Financially, therefore, this system provides a strong incentive to buy time at larger congregated services, where you can buy the most hours for your individual funding plus parental contribution. Parents have to set such a service solution against, perhaps, the more expensive hours of a more individualized service. Community access funding can also be used for access to adult education courses at TAFEs (colleges), which can also, of course, be funded by parents or individuals themselves. Some people combine time at a day centre with a college course. The problem is further compounded, in many STs, by the assessment, at ST level, of people for a 'total package' of accommodation and daytime activity, where the accommodation agency will provide or buy daytime activity in addition to the residential care element of its service. Such a practice naturally increases the amounts being bid for individuals, and therefore similarly increases the number of people who get no funding at all.

This then gets mixed up, as far as parents are concerned, with Commonwealth funding for 'business services', especially since the introduction of 'case-based funding' in all STs, an initiative that sees the money for business services paid to the agency, not directly to the person or family. As from July 2006, a web-based assessment, the Disability Maintenance Instrument (DMI), completed by the business service agency and the family, is adjudicated by the Commonwealth Department of Family, Community Services and Indigenous Affairs (FaCSIA) and reviewed every two years.

There is also confusion on which 'standards' apply to particular services, since these exist at both ST and Commonwealth level, and though they overlap, there is not total harmony between them, and there are different ways of monitoring compliance (Disability Standards Review and Quality Assurance Working Party 1997).

Such confusion contrasts with the positive and hopeful message from the Commonwealth website about how they fund 'a range of employment and related services for people with disability'. This would also tell me about the benefits my offspring would receive through the social security system, known as Centrelink, which body also determines his 'job readiness', and here the first clouds appear on the horizon. The assessment processes for suitability for different sorts of employment services, and also the level of social security payments, can be carried out both by Centrelink itself, via a regional branch, or by 'a local employment service' who may help you to complete the assessment. Here again confusion comes between 'business services', and 'open employment'. For people with intellectual disabilities, the former would be developments from what used to be called 'sheltered workshops', i.e. places that did real work, but on sites that were themselves more or less segregated. This is particularly true of services run by some of the large, multi-state welfare agencies, for whom people with intellectual disabilities are only a small part of their client group, and who provide accommodation and 'community activities' as well as 'business services'. As noted above, funding for business services comes from FaCSIA, a different government source than open employment, whose schemes are funded by the Commonwealth Department of Employment and Workplace Relations (DEWR), and are used more by other disabled groups. In DEWR schemes; the service provider is not the employer, they merely assist people to get open employment, and wages may be according to award rates or as assessed by to DEWR's productivity-based Supported Wage System (SWS). It therefore seems to be in the interests of 'business service' agencies, other things being equal, to have people 'on the books' rather than meet the strict requirements of helping them to achieve totally open employment. The benefit system also gives this incentive, as people working in business services can receive a level of income that will not affect their Centrelink payments, whereas with the minimum wage and other issues in the open employment market, these finances quickly disappear. So, as in Scandinavia, the 'real work' role with a market-based employer has to be set against unrealistic pay rates, an effect noted in Australia some time ago (Tse 1984). On the other hand, even with the degree of correlation between the work role and open employment in the 'business service' of the opening story, the full workplace experience is not there, but a better level of payment is (to both the agency and the person). Only those agencies that either have their sole purpose to find full open employment for people with intellectual disabilities, or who have a sufficiently wide range of services to enable people to move from their business services section to their open employment services are likely not to feel the financial incentive to 'keep people', especially as the move to case-based funding comes into full force. For these services there is still, however, the tension between, as one agency put it 'the provision of supported employment for the disabled employees and the operation of a commercially viable business' (Koomarri 2005: 6).

The overall system of CSTDA, though based on the Disability Services Act, does not give an automatic right to services, and the public and private utterances of politicians and policy-makers continue to emphasize the assumption that parents and carers will need to take a part in the provision of, or payment for, services for their offspring (Croft 2000). In terms of what happens to people in the daytime therefore, my overall impression is of a work-oriented system, but one which has a built-in financial incentive for that work: (1) not to be in the open market; or (2) to be in large segregated sheltered workshops. Some of the places I observed either ignored those incentives, or worked round them, in order to provide activities as close to ordinary work as possible, and in inclusive settings. They seem, however, to be something of a minority. As for those not deemed eligible for 'employment services' (or who have 'chosen' not to seek work – often meaning their parents have chosen this route), the picture is bleaker, with limited funding meaning ever more needy people do not win the 'funding round lottery'. Looking at what happens in residential services, the picture does not get rosier.

Residential services – is the pendulum swinging back?

> Many of the small, personalised services were developed in Queensland around a decade ago. Despite their proven record . . . little support has been given to their sustainability or to any new developments. The excitement and challenge, which people with disabilities and their families felt with the opportunities to create and influence those new ventures, have now gone. With few opportunities for people to get together and funding arrangements not supporting the development of new services, the leadership and creativity that was shown in getting these services up and running are no longer valued. People with disabilities and families are left to do it all alone.
>
> (QPPD 2005: 21)

The words of Queensland parents, though a particularly radical group, set up to some extent in tension with the large, parent-founded, service-providing agency of that State in the 1980s, reflect the picture that I was consistently given in my time in Australia. This was sometimes put even more forcefully, with the word 'crisis' occurring more than once in my notes as I travelled round the country.

Residential care also seems to be the area which still has a significant number of services provided directly by the STs' disability departments. A key part of this provision is a number of the remaining large institutions, which are by no means all closed. Government statistics for disability as a whole (AIHW 2005) still show nearly 4,000 people in 'large institutions' with over a thousand more in 'small institutions' and 'hostels'. This is roughly half the number in 'group homes', but still a sizeable group. The proportion of people in the 'intellectual disability' category for accommodation services, at 54 per cent, is slightly higher than their representation in all services (41 per cent). As well as the large institutions, there are also a significant number of ST-provided care places in group homes, though an equally large number are provided by the bigger, multi-state agencies, mostly from the historical charity sector. As we saw in New Zealand, such group homes, with numbers of residents normally ranging between 4–8 people, were the 'radical' alternative to the institutions in the early days of normalization/SRV, and seem to have become the default option in both countries. The 'small, personalised services' noted in the QPPD report (2005) quoted at the beginning of this section tended to come more in the latter decade of the twentieth century, when the influence of SRV, especially through parent-led initiatives, was at its height (Johnson 1998; Community Resource Unit 2003). Since then, for a variety of reasons, they seem to have remained as examples of what might be achieved, rather than becoming the norm of residential services.

Part of the reason for this state of affairs is the overall welfare funding reforms by Commonwealth and ST governments (Saunders 2005), such that the achievement of any funding at all for accommodation appears to be much more difficult. Commonwealth figures still report over 50 per cent of disabled people living with their parents, and I heard many stories, supported by survey data (Croft 2000: CRU 2003) of desperate parents in their seventies and eighties providing the caring for their 50–60-year-old sons and daughters. As with the funding for day services, of course, this gives a strong incentive to parents to take whatever accommodation is offered, and applications to the 'funding round' become an annual lottery which breeds resentment in the 'losers', with 'winning' meaning achieving funding, rather than careful evaluation of what the funding might buy. The QPPD again put the case powerfully:

> Competition and resentment have been fostered by the current system, with those families or people with disabilities who have funding and those people who have struggled to develop good supports

being seen as the lucky ones. . . . Little new personalised service development has been supported to happen.

(QPPD 2005: 21)

At ST government level, a further consistent story was the tendency for those governments' disability services departments to have fallen prey to the trend towards managerialism, discussed in the previous chapter. The state of Western Australia made a certain name for itself in the 1990s by its system of Local Area Coordinators who, in crude terms, combined the roles of assessor, approver and coordinator of service allocation in that state. These were people with a speciality in disability or intellectual disability, who had often taken a strongly SRV-oriented leadership course at the Centre for the Development of Human Resources at Edith Cowan University in Perth. Other STs followed suit, but it was reported to me that, in recent years, such specialties were being discouraged. With the rise of individualized funding at the same time as budget restraint, the bureaucratic processes to administer the system has, as we saw in New Zealand, become more routinized and anonymous, emphasizing the financial and employment responsibilities of the fundholders (often parents) rather than the sort of life being led by those using the funds.

The move to individualized funding of residential services has had considerable variability across Australia. Those seeking to find an individualized solution need to find both accommodation and an appropriate level of support, and again, agencies offering both are the easier, and cheaper, option for those who achieve funding. Some of the smaller agencies, attempting to be more person-centred, and some parent-led initiatives have attempted to make use of public housing, which comes from the generic housing department of local government, for the accommodation side of the picture. This has offered definite possibilities, but the timing of people getting to the top of the housing list, even with some hastening of the process because of allocations for disability, does not necessarily coincide with the *care* funding becoming available, if it ever does. So then parents have to decide whether to take the housing offer, and somehow subsidize the support, which can result in them having to create their own mini-agency, or miss the housing offer and wait for the care funding, thereby going back down the housing list. QPPD sum up the situation in their state:

> Currently Queensland has no alternative service models where people can have good personalised supports, yet be shielded from these onerous bureaucratic, administrative and legal responsibilities of running the service. This leads to people with disabilities having prescribed and regimented lives with the one approach fitting all. Many people's homes and community based respite centres operate like

small institutions with similar atypical and often abusive cultures and routines. Funding policy is supporting this more and more by promoting mechanisms for people to live together. Residents are expected to fit in with one another, otherwise they are not welcomed and are expected to find a vacancy where they can be placed elsewhere. Therefore ordinary community living is not an option.

(QPPD 2005: 21)

In all the places I visited, therefore, the response to my question about what were the chances of my son leaving home, ranged from 'no chance, because you are not in crisis', through, 'if you buy him the house and employ the staff', to 'if you accept what the system has to offer, then you might get a place in a group home'. The overwhelming impression was that if you are deemed to be coping with your offspring at home, then applications for funding have very little chance. One parent I talked to had been turned down for the fifth time, and the letter from the government instructed them not to apply again 'unless your circumstances change'.

'Non-direct' services – families, money and advocates

Residential services in Australia, as noted, have raised the issue of small-scale 'parent-led' services, which leads back to the broader discussion of the previous chapter, of how far parents should be involved in their *adult* offspring's lives. I visited such a small group in Brisbane, where families combine in a geographically finite neighbourhood. The organization, which needed to be formalized in order to access various funding sources, also clearly needed to involve parents' full agreement, and in fact was based on the notion of parents as a key and continuing part of people's lives. Their objectives, beliefs and assumptions contain many familiar items regarding the lives of their offspring that spring from SRV influences, but one highlights our issue: 'Regardless of capacity or skill, families have a natural authority and are entitled to influence the direction of their son's or daughter's life, if they have remained faithful and committed to that person's development and wellbeing' (Homes West 2005: 11).

Acceptance of that belief can be put under pressure, and be in conflict with others. If, for example, parents feel that their sons or daughters would be better off in an institution, or even a large group home, then a group could well promote such establishments. In addition, the proviso 'if they have remained faithful and committed to that person's development and well being', could be read, and is in other countries, especially the UK, as a moralistic and divisive judgement on parents in terms that are inherently hard to measure (Brookes 1993; Ramcharan et al. 1997). The issue is made more complex in Australia by the pressures on parents, on the one hand, 'to let go', while at the same time being expected to make a major contribution to the care of their offspring. The question is still very much unresolved for me, as will be discussed later when what actually is happening in Adam's life is revealed, but I can certainly sympathize with the Queensland parents in their comments on family influence

> When families make suggestions about providing more appropriate, personalised or responsive supports to meet their family member's needs they get labelled as difficult, rather than considering how the service can be more flexible and do a better job. It is even more rare that people with disabilities themselves are talked with about how they want to live their life. Usually things happen around them and to them rather than with them. In this way the roles that people with disabilities and family members play in directing what happens in life is devalued with workers taking an overly professional stance of knowing what is best.
>
> (QPPD 2005: 23)

So the lesson from those agencies that have done things that seek to provide valued lives for people is that parents need to stay involved, but also that future planning is essential, which brings us to other services that have usually figured in these final sections.

The formal definition of advocacy services for the purposes of the CSTDA states that they are 'designed to enable people with a disability to increase the control they have over their lives through the representation of their interests and views in the community' (AIHW 2005: 12). The CSTDA statistics reveal expenditure under this heading, which also includes information provision, by both STs and the Commonwealth government, though mostly below 1 per cent of total expenditure of STs and around 3 per cent of Commonwealth government spending (AIHW 2005: 6). As far as people with intellectual disabilities are concerned, this funding, with other sources, has helped in some STs to set up family support services. Broader developments, however, putting on national or inter-state events and contributing to publication of accessible and challenging contributions to disability debates have come from the Community Resource Unit (CRU). Based in Brisbane, but reaching many other parts of Australia with their events and publications (CRU 2007), CRU seem especially good at reaching the voices of parents and people with disabilities themselves. They have also been a key part, with many members in common, of the SRV network in Australia, with, as noted, CRU and Values in Action putting on the major series of events presented by Wolf Wolfensberger and his colleagues in 1997. That same visit saw Wolfensberger speaking to a large gathering of advocacy groups from all over Australia, and the concept of Citizen Advocacy, formulated by Wolfensberger in the 1970s, also has a significant presence in Australia.

As a participant in those 1997 events, however, I was taken with the change in the degree of optimism in Australia, from that point to the time of my recent visit, when both the views of CRU members and their publications (e.g. CRU 2005; Shevellar et al. 2005) painted a far gloomier picture than eight years earlier. Particularly in the specific area of intellectual disability, the relative success of the broader disability movement (though far from total – see Goggin and Newell (2005) for a recent analysis) has left many parents and people with intellectual disabilities feeling that they have had their 'day in the sun' in the late 1990s and are now, in the words of the then Director of CRU, tempted 'to give up hope, to speak of lost dreams and resignation, to forecast little improvement in the social conditions for people' (Sherwin 2005: 64).

The fact that they have not done so, nor does Sherwin encourage them to act on that temptation, says much, in my view, for the value base of the individuals and groups involved. New Zealand showed us the issues that arose when the central policy appeared highly values led, but the mechanisms of administration and the presence of one particular supplier of services dominate the agency scene, albeit leaving many more key individuals with a shared vision to hold services to the values of the strategy.

ADAM'S WORLD TOUR

An adult citizen of Australia

As Adam came up to 18, depending on how active we were as parents, and also where we fitted in the income-based class system, then options for Adam would vary. They would vary in detail depending on which ST we were in, but not in broad terms. If we applied for options that might lead to employment in the daytime, we would probably have been advised to go to a local agency that provided 'business options', i.e. sheltered employment with a varying degree of segregation, or, if we were really ambitious, to an agency that would try and find Adam open employment. Employment earnings affecting the means-tested pension, the focus more on people with physical disabilities, and the fairly tight criteria for job placement and retention would make Adam quite a 'high risk' service user of such agencies, however. Agencies that provide *both* business service and open employment assistance might be Adam's best bet, but there are not all that many of those. We would also now have to apply for funding on an individual basis, through an agency, and complete the DMI on-line form which would then determine what sort of funding they would get for him. If we made out that Adam was someone with 'severe needs', we might get funding for 'community options' or we might even get into some of the agencies that still have block grants for these services. They mostly seem to be in segregated groups, though many claim to 'go out' into the community for activities of various sorts. We may get no funding at all, and what happens to Adam in the day would then be up to us to provide, or pay for.

As for leaving home, we would be very unlikely to get funding for Adam as he is in reality, i.e. a competent young man with Down's syndrome. If we were in 'crisis', either because Adam had more severe needs or we just couldn't cope to the point of throwing him out, then funding might be available, but not necessarily for fulltime accommodation or for a personalized living arrangement for Adam. If we wanted that, especially if we still wanted to be involved in Adam's life, we might try to set up a small community service ourselves, but this would depend on our being able to afford the time and money to do this individually, or the ability to get a number of people to join us. Otherwise, it would be easier, if we did get funding or we had the money, to accept a group home 'package' that included daytime activity, and leave Adam to the variable care of the service system. We, and he, might get advocacy support, or information from organizations funded to provide this, to help us search, but might find ourselves as one more in their lists of unmet need on which campaigns are currently proliferating.

Australia seems more devolved than New Zealand, with ST governments having a much greater say in the amount and type of services, but appears less free of national influence than we shall see in Canada and the USA. This means, I think, that the Commonwealth/State tension over payment for services is known about, and exists, across the country, and the relatively small number of STs still enables a *national* network of people to have an influence beyond their home patch. So the question 'who pays – who cares?' does have an *Australian* answer, not just a set of regional ones, though as Adam's world tour box shows, the detail of what he might get would vary somewhat with where in Australia we lived. As we move to the other side of the world, that variation increases somewhat.

6 Canada
Values still to the fore?

'What matters it how far we go' his scaly friend replied.
'There is another shore you know, upon the other side.
The further off from England, the nearer is to France –
Then turn not pale, beloved snail, but come and join the dance.
Will you, won't you, will you, won't you, will you join the dance?
Will you, won't you, will you, won't you, will you join the dance?'

(Lewis Carroll)

INSTANT IMPACTS

Canada – a university student

Arriving after midnight at one of my Canadian locations, my host told me of her concerns about a young woman with Down's syndrome, who had been admitted to hospital following a particularly virulent and sudden cancer. My host, and the circle of friends around the young woman, which included her devoted parents, had been visiting her regularly in the week or so after her admission, and were most concerned about the future. My jet-lagged sleep was briefly disturbed by a telephone ringing at about 4 a.m., and this proved to be the news that the young woman had died in the night. I was to see pictures and hear about her life over the next week, not just those alongside the highly positive obituary that appeared in the city newspaper, but also in the broader information given to me as part of my study. In particular, though this was far from her sole achievement, the young woman was part of a group at the local university that had led the way on inclusive education at that level. She had been one of the leaders of the group, who 'audited' courses, and were able, by mutual consent of the individual class teachers, to undertake modified assignments that were properly evaluated and could gain credits. This sort of group was a feature of both US and Canadian higher education services; far from universal, but present in significant numbers, where inclusion seems to have gone further than some other countries, especially at the tertiary level. For the young woman who so sadly died on my arrival in her city, it certainly represented one of a number of valued roles which she had occupied in her short life, and which, I believe, added to a positive perception of people with intellectual disabilities in that part of Canada, something I was to see elsewhere in the country.

Introduction – back again

Canada and the USA were the two places I had visited most prior to my 2005 study tour, and thus I was already aware, despite many new discoveries, that the provincial variation in services, and the sheer number of service agencies, meant trying to give a precise picture of both countries, especially the USA, was an even more impossible task than the rest of the book. States, in the USA, and Provinces and Territories (PTs hereafter) in Canada have significant government authority, including funding and governance of welfare services. When combined with a market orientation towards welfare in both countries, this makes describing services in one location, let alone the country as whole, very difficult. The even greater difficulty of the USA will be addressed in the next chapter, and my Canadian friends would not forgive me if I bracket the two countries much longer, but it is important to make the point that even a relatively frequent number of exposures to the two cultures and their services still leaves a hazy picture of either.

These chapters will also, as noted earlier, have very little to say about the aboriginal peoples of the two countries, though here I did notice a distinct difference in more recent times between Canada and the USA, but only in broad terms. This relates to ongoing attempts by the Canadian federal government to deal with the historic legacy of the treatment of those of aboriginal descent, in terms of carrying out obligations under various century-old treaties, and attempting to make reparations for certain practices of the colonizers. In terms of distinct intellectual disability services within this group, however, the situation seemed to be much closer to the Australian than the New Zealand experience, in that the issues that faced many people of aboriginal descent were of such an overwhelming nature that separating out such specific services was not a frequently addressed task.

The most fundamental cultural mix, that of the French and English ancestry of the current Canadian population, is obvious to any visitor, not least in its bilinguality. Less obvious superficially, but apparent if one spends any time in Canada, is the much broader range of cultural backgrounds, many giving almost as old a European presence (and languages) as the colonizing pair above, others more recent, but no less numerous, especially people from Asia and the Caribbean. When combined with the vast open spaces of the country, even allowing for the degree of urbanization we noted in Chapter 1, some clues emerge about my impression of intellectual disability services in Canada.

Canada could be said to have often led the world in terms of ideas and values in this field, and resultant service practices, with educational inclusion a prime example, seem to have had a more comprehensive impact across the country than the patchy, if sometimes brilliant, developments in the USA. Equally, the welfare system within Canada, despite PT variation, and though far from the comprehensive coverage of Scandinavia, seems to have generated less of the parental desperation I found in Australia. On the other hand, the dominance of parent-led groups in the innovations of the last decades of the twentieth century seems to have created some major service 'empires'. Provision of what was once radical, especially in residential services, is now commonplace and subject to criticism, and there remains a small but significant minority of people in institutions. In short, the service system in Canada could be compared to its geography, physical and social, with the breathtaking mountain ranges, lakes and rivers alongside vast tracts of flat and featureless plains, and vibrant and cultured modern cities contrasting with struggling traditional rural industries, poverty-ridden native reservations, and issues of urban and racial tension. The history of what the newcomers of the past 250 years have done to the country's much older physical and social environment, with both good and bad results, is matched to a degree by the history of services.

History of services in Canada

Early services – few and far between

The main early developments in Canadian services, as we have seen in the other British colonies, relate strongly to contemporary events in the mother country. PT differences, though their separate responsibility for general welfare was established as far back as the British North America Act of 1867, do not seem to have affected early intellectual disability provision, for the simple reason that very little existed before the turn of the twentieth century. The waves of immigration of that period, often with differing cultural views of disability, the hardship of much of the landscape, and the relatively late industrialization of Canada meant that identification of people with intellectual disabilities by the education system and urbanization were not perhaps as pronounced as in Europe (Laird 2003; Chupik 2004). In addition, the attempts at schooling for the indigenous population in 'residential schools', still the subject of controversy and reparation claims in Canada, took up quite a lot of the attention of pioneering educationalists. In the early decades of the twentieth century, therefore, few service options for parents of children with intellectual disabilities were available. Indeed, there are a number of examples (Broda 2004), of such children either being abandoned by their families at church-run orphanages, or being sent to live with distant relatives, as an extra pair of hands in the basic physical effort to survive in remote communities. Those with more obvious disabilities could, however, end up being institutionalized in psychiatric hospitals or in hospital wards for 'crippled or handicapped' children, and then remaining there as they became adults.

Eugenics and 'mental hygiene'

Discussions on eugenics, already noted, found their way into Canada via the growing professions of medicine, specifically 'mental health', many of whose leaders would have come out from the UK. Equally, however, in broader political and policy-making circles, eugenic ideas were fuelled by the greater awareness of the 'mental health' of the population generated by the 1914–18 war. We have also seen a number of examples in earlier chapters of more powerfully expressed eugenic views in areas dominated by rural and farming interests and their associated politicians, usually expressed in agricultural terms as a concern over the 'decline in the national stock'. Both such influences had their parallels in Canada, exemplified by the formation of the Canadian National Committee for Mental Hygiene (CNCMH), founded by Hincks and Beers in 1918 (Canadian Mental Health Association 2006).

They were soon commissioned by various provinces to look at their facilities, and found that the theoretical distinction between 'mental disease and deficiency', made in the Committee's founding statements, did not often apply in practice, especially in the rural areas. The Committee's findings were sufficiently concerning that they were often reported confidentially to the PT governments. Ironically, one of the institutions visited in Manitoba, which reportedly 'shocked' the inspectors by its conditions in 1918, was, as we shall see later, about to be given a 40 million dollar refurbishment by the Manitoba government at the time of my visit nearly 90 years later (Melnick 2005). The Committee's work, and the growing political impetus of eugenics in the 1920s and 1930s, also increased spending on the hospitals over that period.

The social gospel – state provision for some

At the same time, more general welfare provision was beginning to be influenced by the rise, in a number of PTs, of politicians and parties influenced by what has been called the 'social gospel movement (*The Canadian Encyclopaedia* 2007). Their effect was gradual, but did result, over the decades between the wars, in the introduction of the basic elements of state-provided pensions and publicly funded health care. One politician, J. S. Woodsworth, left the church to lay the foundation for, and become the first leader of, the Cooperative

Commonwealth Federation (CCF), a social democratic party which later became the New Democratic Party (NDP). Another, Thomas Douglas, was Scottish-born, also a Baptist minister, and CCF premier of Saskatchewan from 1944 to 1961, where he led the first socialist government in North America and introduced universal public medicare to Canada. From 1961 to 1971, he led the NDP at the federal level, going on to be voted 'The Greatest Canadian' of all time in a 2004 CBC poll. Interestingly, his 1933 thesis for his MA in Sociology, from McMaster University (Douglas 1933) was on eugenics, proposing a solution to 'the problems of the subnormal family' by sterilizing intellectually and physically disabled Canadians, and sending them to institutions. Changing his views after a trip to Nazi Germany in 1938, however, he apparently rarely mentioned his thesis in later life, and his government never enacted eugenics policies, though two Canadian provinces, Alberta and British Columbia, did enact eugenics legislation in the 1930s.

Douglas' 1933 findings were in keeping with the broader views of the time, of course, partly due to crude assessments, as discussed in other chapters, 'revealing' that the extent of mental disorder was greater than expected, i.e. more people were diagnosed. Following recommendations from such surveys, provincial governments spent over six million dollars on 'improving facilities' over the ensuing couple of decades (McLaren 1990; Canadian Mental Health Association 2006).

As for children, there were effects from growing political pressure to diagnose immigrants in the Depression period, the perceived need for educational improvement of the existing population and the continuing eugenic pressure for 'prevention' as well as 'cure'. Surveys of schoolchildren, conducted by various groups (Laird 2003) again 'revealed' numbers of 'retarded children', leading to either special classes or, more commonly in the urban areas, special 'schools for retarded children' being established by school boards. These sat alongside the existing institutions, such as the Manitoba School for Retardates, which later became the Manitoba Developmental Centre.

Normalization crosses the border

So we have a similar picture, going into the post-war decades, to the countries we have discussed so far. PT-provided or charitable institutions, often taking people as children and leaving them to grow into adults at the institution; sterilization, both in the institutions and at the instigation of parents; and some special classes or special schools for children diagnosed as 'retarded'. It was, again moves from parents, and parents' organizations, that began to change things.

In his account of the development of normalization in North America, Wolfensberger (1999) recalls that he had been approached in 1971 by G. Allan Roeher, head of what was then called the Canadian Association for the

Mentally Retarded (CAMR), to come and work at the Institute on Mental Retardation, a research and publication body sponsored by the Association. Such an invitation reflected Wolfensberger's growing reputation, following the publication of *Changing Patterns* (Kugel and Wolfensberger 1969) as well as the wider debate on normalization generated by that report, and the activities of the small international group noted in Chapter 2. The contribution of Roeher, also from Saskatchewan and the 'social gospel' tradition, was significant. Blanchet (1999: 437–8) describes the key elements that affected services in the early 1970s, revealing the distinctiveness of the Canadian development from its large neighbour to the south, as well as its place in relation to Europe. His views can be summarized as follows:

- A 'vision and a practice of consumer participation' – here Blanchet singles out Roeher, his Saskatchewan roots, and that province's decentralization of its social services, as leading to CAMR trying to establish a network of integrated community services, called COMSERV. Here families would collaborate with local administrations to produce an overall plan for services based on people living in the community.
- The parent association movement developing their role as advocacy for better living conditions, rather than service provision.
- 'Young professional dissidents' – here the normalization and Wolfensberger connection are cited, which we have seen in earlier chapters.
- Canadian traditions of social justice being sympathetic to the development of integrative policies, 'without having recourse to the courts, as was the case in the United States'.

Blanchet's issues are still of relevance today, as is his review of the current situation in 1994. This highlights:

- Much institutional care remaining, with little choice, even in group homes, of where and with whom people live, and a significant movement from institutions to nursing homes.
- Despite great successes, still limited integration in schools.
- Over 80 per cent of people without employment or even 'significant day activity'.
- More than 90 per cent of adults living on income support programmes.
- Little impact nationally of court decisions on rights, despite provincial and national Charters of rights being adopted.
- Continuing social isolation.

Blanchet's view of parents' organizations reverting from service provision to an advocacy and informational role, while it might be true at national or PT level, was less so at more local level. Wolfensberger (1999) notes some hostile reaction to his 1973 paper on the 'stages of evolution of voluntary agencies' in that those who did not want to get out of the service-providing part of the associations (which provided considerably more funds than the advocacy and information side of the business) began to gain or retain control in certain places.

Changing planning decades – changes to the present

The pace of change also did not seem to meet initial hopes. The much vaunted COMSERV projects, as noted at the turn of the decade by Flynn and Nitsch (1980), had taken a long time and much training to get off the ground, moving from a 'Plan for the 1970s' to a 'Plan for the 1980s'. Flynn and Nitsch call this name change 'a somewhat wry comment on the vagaries and torpor of the change process' (ibid.: 379).

Activities begun in Toronto in the early 1970s had continued, however, in terms of leadership and other developments by Wolfensberger on his return to the USA in 1973. This was to see, among other things, the developments of the second and third versions of the PASS instrument, the latter (Wolfensberger and Glenn 1975) subsequently being used worldwide, up to and after the development of its successor PASSING (Wolfensberger and Thomas 1983). These, and the *Normalization* text (Wolfensberger 1972), were not only developed during this time, but NIMR acted as the publishers after some unpromising responses by mainstream academic publishers. So as well as recruiting a group of leaders, not just in normalization but also in the burgeoning field of Citizen Advocacy, and publishing the book that was voted, in 1991, by a panel of experts as the most important in the field (out of 11,300 articles and books reviewed) (Race 2003), the importance of Wolfensberger's time at the NIMR is considerable and it was no coincidence that the first international gathering on *A Quarter Century of Normalization and Social Role Valorization* should have been held in Canada. Blanchet's 1994 review of contemporary issues at that conference (Blanchet 1999), however, shows the limits to progress despite the fervour of the 1970s. In some views, the initial impact of normalization in Canada was not de-institutionalization, but attempts to 'normalize' institutions (L'Institut Roeher Institute 1999). This rather pessimistic view contrasts with other histories of the period, with the situation in Ontario, for example, being described in more immediately progressive terms. One talks of the development, in the 1970s and 1980s of 'a wider range of services to those who were involved in community living as a lifestyle than had formerly been the case, and addressed many, but not all, of the aspects of lifestyle that were being addressed within the institutions' (Buell and Brown 1999: 119).

Once again we come to the paradox of radical developments, much publicized both within and outside Canada, but question marks as to the extent of their implementation on the ground. The 'heady days' did at least, it seems, have some results in terms of the governance of services at PT level, with many PTs following Ontario's example in its Developmental Services Act of 1974. This transferred the responsibility for services in Ontario to people with intellectual disabilities from the Ministry of Health to the Ministry of Community and Social Services, symbolically at least viewing intellectual disability as a social, rather than health, matter. On the ground, however, Ontario was to take a further 13 years to produce 'a long range strategy for deinstitutionalization' (Ministry of Community and Social Services 1987) and Buell and Brown (1999) report that even this has only been partly achieved.

Other examples reprise the points Blanchet made in 1994, and we shall see that radical developments that he cites as hope for the future, such as inclusive education, all forms of advocacy, and the development of parent groups not providing direct services, but campaigning, all maintain strong roots in Canada. Many of them, though far from all, stem from the group of leaders developed during Wolfensberger's time at Toronto, others from subsequent movements such as the more general disability rights movement. We will also see, however, as we move on to the overview and then detailed impression of Canadian services, that many of Blanchet's more negative points about the 1994 situation still hold good 12 years later.

Services in Canada – an impression

Overview – provincial governance

Table 6.1 reveals the PTs as the main source of funding of most services, and PT governance of *access* to services, though *provision* is largely through agencies, with the key exception of schools and certain health-related services. Federal funding is largely confined to direct financial payments of disability pensions, though they have over the years (not revealed in Table 6.1) provided earmarked funding for specific initiatives. We should also note again the role of parent-led groups in Canada, not just in the formation of provincial and national 'Associations for Community Living', but more local branches too, many of whom are major service providers.

This, too, is a significant part of the paradox that is my lasting impression of the services in Canada. Details of the different levels then follow.

Pre-natal services – Canadian freedom

As a general statement, it can be said that abortion in Canada is not limited by law (Wikipedia 2006). Social pressures, campaigning by pro-life groups and other non-legal obstacles exist, of course, but Canada appears to be one of only a small group of nations who do not place legal restrictions on abortion, with

Table 6.1 Schematic overview of 'services' that affect the lives of people with intellectual disabilities in Canada

'Service'	Formal organizational place	Specialist or generic?	Main source(s) of funding
Pre-natal services	Provincial/local hospitals and health centres Medical practices Private hospitals and practitioners Screening clinics	Generic and specialist	PT Health departments Health Insurance
Post-natal and early childhood services	Provincial/local hospitals and health centres Medical practices Private hospitals and practitioners Early childhood agencies, some voluntary	Generic clinical services, but agency input varying in specialization	PT Health departments Health Insurance Provincial Children and family departments- generic or Developmental Disability sections
Non-educational services for children	Agencies, including those providing respite services Local Associations for Community Living (ACLs)	Specialist and generic	PT Children and family departments- generic or Developmental Disability sections Charitable funding – e.g.United Way
Education services – children and young adults	Local School Boards Independent school trusts	Generic and specialist	PT Education department funding to Local School Boards – some PTs also use local property taxes to fund schools
Education services – adults	Colleges and Universities	Generic and specialist	General tertiary education funding
Residential services – adults	Agencies – some Provincial direct provision Some public housing	Generic and specialist	Provincial funding via individual or block grants to agencies – not mandatory
Daytime services – non-work	Agencies- some Provincial direct provision	Largely specialist	Provincial funding via individual or block grants to agencies – not mandatory

Daytime services – work	Agencies, either supported employment or open employment or both	Largely specialist	Provincial funding via individual or block grants to agencies – not mandatory
Leisure assistance	Agencies – usually as part of broader package	Largely specialist	Provincial funding via individual or block grants to agencies – not mandatory
Advocacy services	Agencies, including parent support agencies, individual Citizen advocacy agencies, and campaigning organizations	Specialist	Provincial funding via individual or block grants to agencies – not mandatory Charitable funding
Financial assistance	Federal Social Assistance	Specialist within generic service	Federal tax credits and Social Assistance
Parental 'support services'	Acting as all parents Also setting up individual or community agency	Specialist, in that all children are different	Own finances, or individual funding for specific parent-led initiatives

access to such services among the easiest in the world. Over 110,000 abortions are performed in Canada every year, with around 90 per cent performed in the first trimester, and only 2–3 per cent performed after 16 weeks (Wikipedia 2006). The Canadian courts, given this freedom of control, have adopted the position that a foetus is not considered a person under Canadian law until birth. The freedom of individual Canadian citizens, the diversity of the population, and the range of political views across the provinces seem to have ensured no dominance by religious or ideological groups, with most of the current arrangements being a response to the moves for reproductive rights of the 1960s and 1970s, with considerable influence from the USA, though without their backlash from the religious right.

In terms of the specific pre-natal screening of disabled children, therefore, the issue appears not to be one of law, but of availability and access to medical services. As in Australia, Canada has a basic welfare state in terms of health services, covered by the public insurance system known as Medicare, but a great many people have private or employment-based health insurance in addition to this. Testing for conditions such as Down's syndrome is commonplace, though in some clinics these are not paid for by the basic healthcare system, but overall there appears to be a similar basic standard of pre-natal care.

The debates on screening and abortion on the grounds of disability also go on, however, and the general disability movement has been active in these debates. The issue has been clouded to some extent, as in other countries, by that movement also containing a significant number of people coming from a feminist perspective on reproductive rights, and thus in general agreement with the overall abortion freedoms, while at the same time opposing the messages sent by abortion on the grounds of disability (Frazee 2000).

The impression from my discussions with people in Canada, including parents, pretty much bears out the relative weights of the different positions, but, not for the last time in this chapter, it appeared to me that organized lobby groups, especially those originally or currently from the ranks of parents and carers, have a greater chance of getting their views heard than in some of the other countries.

Early childhood services

As we saw in the overview, nearly all services are administered by PTs with different governments deciding on the precise organizational structures and legislation to cover services in their part of the country. The impression I received, however, was that in the early years after birth there is a fairly consistent *generic* child welfare system across the country, though some specialist parts for disabled children are more variable. Issues of *specific* services and their support for children with intellectual disabilities, apart from those with additional physical impairments, seem to come more as the child reaches school age. For those with multiple disabilities, the availability of *physical* care seems adequate, if not plentiful. As with all comments on Canada, however, and even more so the USA in the next chapter, the degree of poverty of parents puts a rider on the foregoing, as does whether they are from the indigenous population. This is not just talking about extreme poverty, but people who have no extra health insurance. The main supports that people in the early years seem to require are financial ones, as we shall see below, though respite care is also an issue, and this creates a double blow to families with no health insurance. After the birth of a child with intellectual disabilities, services from a public health nurse, whose titles vary, are usually covered by PT funding, but many of the specialists need referral and a waiting list, for those not insured, though serious health problems involving hospitalization do come under government schemes.

The national Participation and Activity Limitations Survey (PALS) of all disability groups supports the view regarding finances, and reveals financial effects are felt in a number of areas of life. For example, the average income of a family with a disabled member was 86.2 per cent of the income of family without disabilities; in 62 per cent of all families with disabilities, parents' work was affected by the fact; and in 75 per cent of cases of those who need assistance, parents were reported as needing more help with family responsibilities than they were getting (Statistics Canada 2001).

The issues are not all about money, however. In the same survey, approximately 20 per cent of parents of pre-school children with disabilities report that their child has been refused daycare or babysitting services due to their condition, with the percentage not varying significantly between children with 'mild to moderate' and 'severe to very severe' disabilities. Access to advice, and sometimes advocacy, also seems to be a key issue in whether parents take advantage of possibilities for PT-funded respite care. There is therefore, as Adam's World Tour box indicates, somewhat variable, though at least basic, support for families of pre-school children in Canada. As we shall see below, on the arrival of children at school age, the financial concerns lessen to a degree, as does the effect on parents' employment, but other pressures take over.

ADAM'S WORLD TOUR

Conceived in Canada – what next?

The free availability of abortion provides an interesting contrast with the much higher profile of debate about disability issues, and so the chances of Adam being born were he conceived in Canada depends a lot on who we, as his parents, were, and where we lived. If we lived, like most people, in the great cities, and if we were at least on a middle income, then the chances of our getting tests (possibly via personal or employment health insurance) would be high, but so would our being informed by other groups about disability issues. If we were poor, or newly arrived immigrants in the cities, then it would be more a matter of chance whether we were offered tests, but there would also be more professional pressure to abort if we had a 'negative' result. If we were in the rural areas, especially if we were from the indigenous population, testing would be even more haphazard, but there may well be less pressure.

If Adam were born, then again who we were, and where we lived, would be important. In addition to our income and health insurance, our ability to access advocacy and/or advice from agencies such as the local Association for Community Living would affect whether we received more than just the basic post-natal support from professionals such as a public nurse. If Adam had additional physical or health problems, this would be more likely to occur regardless, and might also include 'respite' care in our own home or some form of unit. Otherwise we would be entitled to financial support, though limited, and would be left to look for advice and support via the above agencies and the local offices of the PT intellectual disability department. This would include advice regarding schooling, and might involve some pre-school developmental input. All of the above would be more accessible if we had money to pay privately and the persistence to demand our 'rights'

Education – inclusion rights, and inclusion realities

In an interesting report, Michael Bach, executive vice-president of the Canadian Association for Community Living, reflects, as he did in a conversation with me when I met him in Toronto, on the 're-thinking' that a number of people in Canada are carrying out, with regard to various aspects of 'radical' developments in the intellectual disability world:

> The rights-based approach to citizenship has given children and adults with disabilities and their families a claim to press on the state to challenge the abuse, poverty and exclusion from education that so many face. We have largely been getting what we asked for in terms of human rights instruments, but people are still excluded.
>
> (Bach 2002: 10)

We have, so far, seen attempts by both national governments (in the case of the first three countries) and national/ST governments in Australia, to bring about a policy of inclusion within their school systems. In the Scandinavian countries, with the total dominance of the welfare state, such practices could be, and were, enforceable by the command process of state education. In Australia and New Zealand, especially the former, the combination of semi-autonomous school boards and the greater preponderance of independent schools seems to have resulted in more variable success, but with inclusive possibilities still there, given (1) persistence; (2) being in the right place; and (3) the presence of support groups or advocates. What I did not detect as a frequent force, though technically it exists and has been used in all those countries, is the resort to law to achieve inclusion. What Bach's comments illustrate for me is the tendency, powerful in Canada but even more so in the USA, for welfare policy, in intellectual disability and elsewhere, to be the result of 'rights' cases. Bach (2002) goes on to give his reasons why he believes such approaches have not resulted in full inclusion, and these can be broadened beyond his focus on education.

First, the ironic but inescapable fact that, in order to define 'rights' for particular groups, societies have to define who is 'entitled' to them, and in the case of disability this involves defining an 'excluded' group as such, in order for them to be 'included', thus labelling and institutionalizing differences. Second, enforcement tends to be through individuals seeking compensation for discrimination. This does not automatically create policy change, but does create antagonistic forces, and can even be factored in, as 'acceptable losses' by systems that do not want to undergo fundamental change. Third, as Wolfensberger (2002) has also pointed out, just as rights can be afforded by societies through legislation, they can be taken away, and the much more powerful local politics of both Canada and the USA means that legislation can usually be altered at that level much more quickly than national legislation, as well as being interpreted in specifically local ways to fit particular political agendas. It is an irony that the 'freedom' brought about, especially in Canada, by the (literal as well as cultural) space for people of differing views and original cultures to live together, also seems to hinder the sort of consensus on *policy*, as opposed to 'rights', that leads to effective practice. 'Choice', the great watchword of many rights activists, and present in nearly every 'mission' or 'vision' statement, *is* what most Canadians have in abundance. Certainly more than many of their vulnerable groups, whose denial of choice is a key element in devaluation and oppression, but being given the 'right to choose' from a set of devaluing options does not make them any more valuing.

We will return to the 'rights' point again, but now go back to our thoughts on education and children with intellectual disabilities in Canada. In 1989, prior to my two-year 'masochistic sabbatical' as a primary school teacher described in the Introduction, I attended the second 'Summer school on Inclusive education' at McGill University, Montreal. With presenters from all over Canada and the USA, including Judith Snow, John McKnight, the late Herb Lovett, and John O'Brien, the event gave a powerful impression of inclusive education in both the USA and Canada, borne out by the continuing major contribution of many participants and leaders through 'Inclusion Press International' (see http://www.inclusion.com/) and elsewhere. There appeared to be far more progress than I had observed in the UK, which we were beginning to experience in practice as Adam came up to 5. What a number of observers have said to me since, or have written about (O'Brien and Forest 1989; McKnight 1996; Hansen 2006) is that, in one respect, those *were* major years of achievement in both countries, especially Canada, in terms of achieving not only rights to inclusion, but the development of techniques and attitudes among, most importantly, teachers. The fact that, 15 years later, comments such as Bach's are still commonplace does not, in my view, represent a failure on the part of that movement, but more a realistic assessment of the complexity and limitations of inclusion, as well as the broader trends affecting education, such as the neo-liberal economic agenda and its accompanying managerialism that we have discussed already.

So how does this paradox of widely acclaimed pioneering approaches existing alongside the same basic issues as all the other countries play itself out in Canada? Reminding ourselves of PT autonomy, and thus variability, over funding, policy and administration, further devolution comes for school-based education in that it is run by local district school boards, covering a geographic area defined by population. Members of these boards are elected but are not usually from the large political parties. Most boards, following the debates of the last decades of the twentieth century, have inclusive policies, and in many cases a 'local school' policy operates, i.e. the normal practice is for children to be offered places at their local school. Within this overall policy, however, there is considerable emphasis on freedom of parents to choose schools that fit other criteria they may have, especially those from a particular religious denomination. Such a situation, however, is less contentious than it might sound, with the range of religions in the different provinces being accommodated somewhat more successfully than is the case in, for example, the UK. As with the issue of language, Canada seems to be able to manage difference in this respect with a degree of tolerance unusual in the modern world.

So much so (relatively) inclusive, and as we have seen, there are a number of examples of good practice (Shaw 1990). Pressures of a broader kind, however, have meant that fewer schools moved through the full spectrum from physical inclusion, via inclusion in some classroom activities (assimilation), to a fully inclusive curriculum (Lutfiyya 2005). Academic assessment in Canada, like Scandinavia, tends to be carried out mostly by schools themselves, or at least on a PT-wide basis, as opposed to the national testing and school league tables of other countries such as the UK. There is therefore greater scope for the curriculum to be varied and created for inclusion, but equally for it to be divided into, within the same school, 'special programmes', i.e. separate segregated programmes for groups with intellectual or other disabilities. This appears to happen less at elementary schools (taking ages roughly 5–11/12-year-olds) but increasingly so through middle and high schools. Teaching aides can come with pupils assessed as needing such support, though there is a debate over their role and whether they are there for the person only, or as an aide to the classroom teacher to create an inclusive class (Andrews and Lupart 2000). There appear to be few segregated 'special schools' for people with intellectual disabilities, though these still exist for other disabled groups, and, as elsewhere, a growing pressure exists for separate facilities for 'autistic' children.

Middle and high schools offer their pupils a 'menu' of courses, from which they are theoretically able to choose any, but the normal core subjects such as mathematics and English are needed for pupils to graduate from high school. Most graduate at 18, though a number who are unlikely to achieve their certificate, especially from some minority and indigenous groups, tend to 'drop out' just before this age, or to have been diverted into some form of vocational route. People with intellectual disabilities, ironically, tend to go on to 21, initially thought of as a 'success' by the inclusion movement, but increasingly being seen as 'warehousing' until 21, because adult services will not always take over until then.

Speaking to a member of a community college that trained staff to work at a front line level in all services, an increasingly common destination for their graduates appeared to be as teacher aides. Her observations of practical placements for her students in these roles confirmed the picture of inclusion painted above. Most schools she had visited had pupils with intellectual disabilities on site but in segregated classes – even an example she gave of an exception to this, where a special education trained teacher was trying to include people in her class, had ended up with inclusion in the 'easy' subjects like Music and Physical Education. So Adam, as his next box indicates, would again have a varied set of chances in education services in Canada.

ADAM'S WORLD TOUR

Going to school in Canada

As we saw in the previous box, school options depend a lot in Canada on whether we, as parents, had been in touch with the service system; which PT we were in and whether we were in a rural or urban part of it; our income and insurance status; and our use of the potential support of advocacy and/or agencies such as the local ACL. Adam's pre-school programmes and then his entry into the school system would therefore also vary according to those factors, but with at least a common assumption of local schooling and physical inclusion being adopted by most School Boards, who ultimately determine what goes on in the school system.

The degree of full inclusion of Adam would then depend on the age level of the school, with more happening at elementary level; possibly whether we wanted a particular religious denominational school; and again whether we were in a rural area, with choice being more restricted. The restriction of choice, however, in the rural areas, can be used to *ensure* inclusion, since the number of children with intellectual disabilities will not normally be sufficient to justify a separate class or unit.

As Adam went through middle and high school, perhaps staying until he was 20/21, he would probably be offered an increasingly separate curriculum, often accompanied by a separate class base as well, but there are many places where separation would not be as pronounced. If the school worked seriously on finding employment for its likely non-graduates, Adam might get some work experience, but would more likely emerge either unknown to adult services, or if we pushed and got in with agencies, lined up for a place in day services. As we shall see, this can include the possibility of employment, and schools in some places facilitate the transition well – others would 'warehouse' Adam until he could be passed on to the service system.

Daytime services – once again, what is work?

The number of positive service examples I saw in Canada, and had seen on previous visits, could easily lead one to suggest a distinct difference from those countries we have seen so far. Talking with people involved with such services, however, and with others, including government officers, many of the familiar issues return. No more so than on the issue of employment, where, more than any of the countries in terms of the quantity and quality of real, paid, work finding schemes, I saw good models in Canada. On the other hand, despite their greater frequency, such schemes were still very much in the minority, and the distinction between their practice and what went on in other 'daytime activity', including the still occurring 'packages' where all of a person's life is governed by the agency providing the accommodation service (including the remaining large institutions, of which more later) was considerable. To this we must again add the greater degree of local autonomy both within and between PTs.

We have seen already that a number of children will have come to the attention of their PT before or during their time at school, possibly even receiving respite services. Apart from estimates of numbers for planning purposes, however, detailed knowledge of *individual* young people with intellectual disabilities attending school is not normally kept by PT service funders for adult services, even as the children come up to school-leaving age. Adult services should, in theory, be involved in transition planning, and liaise with schools, especially if work is a real possibility, but also to prepare a person for what is coming after school. In practice, though PTs may make estimates of the numbers of people coming out of school, and encourage parents to contact them prior to leaving school, individual transition seems to be mostly left to schools, parents, advocates and support agencies. Once a person reaches a certain age (18 in some PTs, 21 in others), they can be referred (usually by parents, though some will have agency help if they are bidding for a specific sort of service) to the PT adult service system. If people are already known to the disability services, this will be effectively a re-referral to the adult part of the system. Regardless of what they are formally called, the workers who then deal with individual people are effectively 'case managers', with caseloads, I was told by both officials and outsiders, of around 100–150 cases at any one time. Before this will have come a determination (or confirmation if they are already known) of whether the individual is eligible, which depends on PT-defined criteria. The PT case manager will then set up a meeting where details of individual and family needs can be formed into a plan, with decisions on funding depending on the match between those needs, available services, and the budget limitations of the case manager or their superior. Such a plan may take a variety of forms and degrees of formality, but the official position is of access to all the services, once eligibility is established.

Budgets are usually set for a finite range of options that have known charges attached, and most of the agencies that may already be involved in a bid will be known to the department. In all my discussions it was acknowledged that accommodation was harder to budget for and allocate than daytime activities, with one commissioner, who had previously specialized in this aspect, holding the view that pressures from activists were for more work and less segregated workshops. This had resulted in some workshops closing, and, as well as agencies finding people 'real work', a number of others were simply 'occupying people', not in real work, but in 'community activities'. Here we are back to the debate that has arisen in each chapter about 'meaningful occupation' vs. 'real work' vs. 'segregation' though with the additional issue, in rural communities, of limited resources meaning that a 'one stop shop' service applies, usually a segregated sheltered workshop.

With some significant exceptions, day and residential programmes tend to be mostly with separate agencies, and parents, especially if advised by support agencies such as ACLs, tend to get connected with 'daytime' agencies before school leaving, so as to approach the PT with a costed package. As we have seen, however, local ACLs vary in terms of whether, and to what degree, they provide direct services themselves, and therefore are in a position of conflict of interest. If they adopt the position of the national Canadian Association for Community Living (CACL), or most provincial offices, then employment is definitely a preference, but in some locations parents (who still have a significant presence in many ACLs) have a loyalty to the sheltered workshops they set up as the daytime alternative to the institutions. In others the ACL, or other organizations founded by parents, may be a major provider of all kinds of services, including 'total packages'.

In a discussion document setting out a 'long-term vision' for services, the national CACL propose that the employment rate of Canadians with intellectual disabilities be increased 'by over 50 per cent' (CACL 2005: 7). The fact that they are calling for an increase *by*, rather than *to* 50 per cent, and that this comes under the heading of achieving 'Employment Equality', reinforces the point, as does the fact that such a goal is at the edge of the time range of the various goals, to be 'achieved by 2015'. Again, however, the fact that the national CACL is raising the issue publicly indicates the Canadian paradox of high awareness struggling to match its ideals in practice.

Two agencies from the same city, both influenced by SRV, provide an example of a radical approach, but the fact that they were in a minority supports the above point One had two programmes adopting a new angle to employment. The first sought, as a general notion, to prepare the *employing community* to welcome people with intellectual disabilities, in fact, 'recruiting a pool of employers'. By dedicating an employee, not to work directly with individuals but to 'market' people with intellectual disabilities as a *workforce*, the agency seemed to have built up a significant number of potential employers. This then complemented their approach with individual people with intellectual disabilities, which involved working with them on their *general* employability, with detailed work on CVs, interview training, etc., rather than preparing them for a particular job. This agency also ran what was effectively an employment project for people while they were still at school, going from the view that ordinary teenagers get into the world of work through evening and weekend working, therefore not taking time out of school. Traditional 'work placements' organized by schools tended (1) to take time away from people being at school, therefore leading to their gradual separation from the education system and (2) to be largely directed at the 'included' group of young people with intellectual disabilities, so that their introduction to the world of work differed from others. The youth project recruits (and pays) young teenagers as mentors, to work with the students with intellectual disabilities, on the sorts of jobs that most teenagers get to supplement their finances while still at school. So employers get a 'package' of two people, with the intellectually disabled person getting paid by the employer, and the mentor by the agency, PASC (2007).

The second agency, from the same city, but much larger and originating in a parents' organization of the 1970s, provided an interesting alternative in employment finding, but as part of its overall approach to the range of services it provided. This is 'roles based planning' described as 'a thoughtful approach to social inclusion AND empowerment' (Ramsey 2005: 2) with their emphasis highlighting what has been seen as a potential tension between the two elements. The broader theoretical issues of this approach will not be discussed here, though they are included in an interesting set of reflections on roles by O'Brien (2005), which cites some quantitative data from the agency. On employment, they note the following, after three and a half years of the new approach:

- Increasing competitive employment rates from 35 per cent to 68 per cent;
- Increasing the average hourly wage from $5.17 to $7.56;
- Increasing the range and perceived societal value of employment roles held by people we support.

(Ramsay 2005: 16)

This picture of innovation in direct employment finding services continued in other provinces, though, as with the above city, the response to my questioning would run as follows. A couple of agencies majoring in employ-ment finding; others totally workshop-based; some involved in 'individual day programmes', i.e. a worker to help people 'do what you want in the day', which can vary considerably, from genuine attempts at meaningful activities to 'bus therapy' (sometimes referred to equally critically as 'mall therapy'). More rural areas, as we have noted, were said to have just one workshop, and only one or two agencies operating services.

Again, the place where individuals end up, whether in a rural or urban area, seems to depend more on the efforts of parents and/or agency/advocacy support than specific levels of 'need'. This will be a major feature of the next section.

Residential services – beyond group homes to 'welcoming communities'?

Although I have visited Canada many times over the years, events that occurred in the relatively short duration of my visit in 2005 illustrate, espe-cially when it comes to accommodation, the paradox of the prominence of radical views co-existing with institutional practices. As noted in the history section, my arrival in Winnipeg coincided with the Manitoba government announcing that one of the two institutions in or near that city would be getting a 40 million dollar refurbishment, amid much controversy. The other institution, in Winnipeg itself, had been reducing but then had to take over most of the hundred or more people from an agency that had been convicted of running a major fraud. In the same week, the national CACL were preparing to be key witnesses in a court case in Ontario, this time on the side of the province, who wished to close one of the few remaining institutions, but were being sued by a parents' lobby to prevent this happening. In both these prov-inces, however, I also visited or heard of small innovative housing projects, some strongly influenced by SRV. A similar contrast came in Alberta, where I was to be shown both what was effectively an institutional campus, though based in a residential area, and told of the other provincial institution, located in a totally rural area some 40 miles from Calgary. Yet, in the same city, I met and heard of individuals with their own homes, jobs, and widely ranging life experiences, and in the same province, a highly respected programme of work with parent groups that kept radical issues at the forefront of discussion.

So the picture continues. At the same time as they were preparing for their day in court, the CACL were publishing the discussion document referred to above, and proposing, among their nine 'benchmarks for achievement', the following

2. Close Institutions and Assure a Home in the Community

• By 2007, there will be no new admissions to large institutions.

- By 2010, all large institutions for persons with intellectual disabilities will be closed.
- By 2013, the number of persons with intellectual disabilities living in inappropriate settings such as long-term care facilities, nursing homes, personal care homes and/or seniors facilities will be reduced by over 50 per cent of its current level.
- By 2015, all supported living environments for persons with intellectual disabilities will be designed and bound by the principles of choice, self-determination and individualized funding.

(CACL 2005: 4)

The need, still, to refer to *admissions* to institutions, let alone their closure, as being targets for two and five years acknowledges their presence, but also their decline. More worrying is the goal with regard to what are effectively institutional alternatives to formally designated institutions, and that the goal is for a reduction, not an elimination of 'inappropriate settings'. Canada are not alone in this, of course, and my impression is that the more the service system is both market-driven and variable within different parts of a country, the more such practices seem to go on. This also applies to the way in which individual funding is regarded. In Scandinavia, it does not appear to have been considered necessary, given the state provision of services, and in New Zealand and the UK it seems to be only on an 'experimental' basis. Australia, on the other hand, seemed to be moving strongly in that direction, with mixed results. While it can produce highly original and individual solutions for people, it can also be a way of effectively barring access to services, if the budgets are limited, and/or putting the burden of both organizing the support system, and contributing to its cost, onto parents. In Canada, it seems to be in favour with CACL and those at the radical end of things, but the power of some of the large-scale providers of services, including local ACLs, tends to make them a large presence in the market when parents look to spend their individual funding. Currently, there tends to be a range of per diem rates that agencies can propose to the PT funders, partly dependent on individual support needs, but also on the agencies' ability to persuade their respective PTs that such support is needed, and the ability or desire of PTs to adjust their rates over time. One province I visited had not adjusted its rates for five years.

So if housing is required, then parents tread a number of complex paths, and success often depends on agencies either having a place vacant, or building up a case for independent living and being granted funding. Generally it seems to take a good while to get placed in an accommodation service, more so if an individual solution is sought, but once there, the place is usually fairly secure. It also seems that who you know, your parents, and the particular provincial caseworker you get determine a lot of things initially, and then the continuing ability of agencies to maintain their original values and focus when faced with competition from larger (and often cheaper) agencies, and shrinking provincial budgets. This is summarized in the final Adam's World Tour box.

ADAM'S WORLD TOUR

An adult citizen of Canada

As Adam came up to 18, or perhaps 21 if we were in certain places, then options would vary considerably. If he had been in the vocational programmes in his school, and if we, as active parents, had already been in touch with agencies, then possibilities of employment could be raised. If this were pursued, he might be funded, assuming he passed the PT eligibility criteria, for time with an employment finding agency. If we did not specifically pursue employment, the most common option for the daytime, again depending on our PT, and how rural a part of it we lived in, would be a sheltered workshop. As for moving out, it would again depend on our ability to push, and Adam's assessed needs, but there would be the chance, in some places, of individualized funding to organize accommodation of Adam's choosing, and with whom he wished to be. More likely would be a small group home, though if his impairments or behaviour were more serious, especially if we found it hard to deal with the system, then larger residential care institutions might be provided. A total 'package' involving the whole of Adam's time, might also be what was worked out, with varying implications for what Adam did during the day, and a variety of possibilities, from institutions to individual apartments, for where he lived. Advocacy assistance for us and Adam might well be forthcoming from our local ACL or other parent networks, but the ACL might also be a large service provider who would tend to steer us towards use of their services, with varying results. Adam himself, again in certain places, might have more of a say in all this, but we as parents would be certainly consulted, and in some places given almost total control, over what was proposed for Adam. If we chose to be part of it, we could probably find a fairly radical parents' group in most urban areas, though we might find ourselves in conflict with others, sometimes to the point of legal action to preserve local facilities of a type that the national ACL, or our radical group, might wish to see disappear.

Who works in services – Canada as a lead to a general discussion

I have noted above my conversation with a person who had taught for many years at a community college. This conversation confirmed information from agency managers and ACL personnel on the wider issue of staff training and qualification.

When her college course was first taught, there was a mandatory placement in institutions but now the college try to get students some placements with families, though group homes and sheltered workshops form the majority. Also, however, as we have seen, because 30 years ago children with intellectual disabilities did not go to mainstream school, support staff were not required, but now school is the most common children's placement for staff in training. There has also been a change in the sort of people coming on the college course. Initially sent by agencies, the college then began taking regular cohorts of new immigrants, people who did something in services as high school work placements, and occasionally but regularly a person who was not working in the field but had an interest, such as an intellectually disabled family member. Teaching has gone from an emphasis on medical and behaviour modification issues to SRV and inclusion, but there are still a number of basic college and other educational requirements, so the course could not be described as all radical material.

An agency CEO from a different province had worked, straight from a psychology degree but with no experience of intellectual disability, in various roles in her agency, including the 'front line'. Because of the size of her particular organization, 'home managers' also tended to be on the front line, and home workers were now taking a similar course to the above at their local community college, then going on to be home managers. She described her front-line workers as generally young, with a high turnover, as agency wages were only just above the minimum wage, and 'fairly minimal' was her view of most agency training. Since inspection of homes seems largely based on physically measurable variables, the qualifications of staff do not figure as an issue. Discussion with a local ACL confirmed that most managers at CEO level have been through university, but not necessarily in social work or disability studies. College courses were helping, and more middle managers were getting involved – as were some from certain agencies on the regular SRV courses in that particular city – but training was not well funded by the province, and agencies were limited in the resources they could give to it.

This picture was similar to my observations in Australia and New Zealand, with very few front-line staff of agencies having significant qualifications, and managers rarely having specific qualifications in intellectual disability. It also appeared to be the case in the USA, and to a large extent in the UK, though the anomalous place of a specialist nursing qualification is still in force there.

So here we have another key difference between the Scandinavian countries and the rest, and it seems to be highly correlated, again, with the extent of the welfare state in those countries and also with the greater emphasis on vocational education at school level. A common response *outside* Scandinavia to my question, 'What sort of qualifications do people need to work here?' was a variant on 'standing upright' or 'a warm pulse'.

'Non-direct services' – part of the system?

In my conversations in Canada, most people who had been around for a period of 20 years or more usually said that positive things had been achieved in their time – the closing or downsizing of many institutions, the greater presence of people in communities. 'Non-direct services', apart from basic financial benefits, which stem from the federal government and have roughly matched those in other countries, could be said to be a significant part of these changes, with small, parent-led services, the greater say of parents over proposals for their offspring, some significant citizen advocacy, and good efforts by certain leaders to mobilize families.

Attempts to develop services began with parents fighting to get anything at all – this seems to have been won on many fronts, with the push from many groups for 'better services'. There are still, as we have seen, some remaining skirmishes over institutions but the battle lines are more difficult to draw up precisely over day programmes and school inclusion after the basic physical integration of such services. So far, so familiar, but the interesting possibility, raised by CACL but also by a number of people in the more radical services, I described in my notes as 'campaigning to develop community'. This is not just about awareness, though I saw a really positive example in the 'Everybody Belongs' campaign in Calgary (http://www.everyonebelongs.com/background.htm) that was not at all about services, but about people being part of communities. Beyond 'community awareness', however, the notion of getting communities 'pulling in' people by demanding their presence, rather than just tolerating it, or worse, is what I perceive to be behind radical, 'non-direct service' moves in Canada. The phrase used by the CEO of the national CACL was 'You can't push a rope – you have to pull with it'. In my view, Canadian society lends itself rather more to this notion than most, with its tradition of independent sub-groups and self-sufficient neighbourhoods. Again, this may be another example of interesting ideas getting an airing in Canada, with the risk of reality falling far short, and the impact of globalization and consumerism is as powerful in Canada as elsewhere, especially given their neighbour across the border. However, the CACL have begun to do some work on what was described as the 'latent desire of communities' – related to the ideas of 'social capital' (e.g. Coleman 1988; Putnam 2000; Fine 2001) which may bear fruit. Those ideas have also, of course, surfaced in the USA but as we shall see in the next chapter, so have many others, not all as hopeful.

7   The United States of America
Freedom to roam the jungle?

Beware the Jabberwock, my son!
The jaws that bite, the claws that catch!
Beware the Jubjub bird, and shun
The frumious Bandersnatch!

                                   (Lewis Carroll)

INSTANT IMPACTS

USA – a third generation of inclusive education

Syracuse, New York State, is known within the worldwide normalization and SRV network as the location of Wolf Wolfensberger's Training Institute, and also the Center for Human Policy (now the Center for Human Policy, Law and Disability Studies) currently led by Professor Steven Taylor, through which many of the 'names' of the radical end of disability academia have passed, or are still involved. None of these people would be known to the beautiful 4-year-old boy with Down's syndrome whom I met on a visit to Jowonio School in Syracuse. I had seen a number of 'inclusive education' settings before, not least during Adam's progress through the English system, and though Jowonio was an impressive example of a 'pre-school' inclusive setting, with the 4-year-old being totally involved with what was going on for all children, yet able to shine out with his own personality, its impact on me came when I discovered that the school had been operating in this fashion for three generations. Attending a PASSING workshop the following week, I noticed, at the beginning of the PASSING manual, thanks to Jowonio School for acting as a pilot location. Factors that will require far more nuanced discussion in this chapter were raised by people at Jowonio; the proximity to Syracuse University, with both academics and students on placement near at hand; the fact of it being a private school, with somewhat limited access for poorer parents despite the school's best intentions; and the subsequent tensions with the local and State education system. Despite this, however, for the school, and more importantly the values behind it, to have lasted the 25 years of turbulence in education in the USA, says something, I believe, for the enduring nature of those values. The young man, who said hello with his eyes, brought tears to mine.

Introduction – return to Disneyland

In a fascinating book, *Jesus in Disneyland* (2000) David Lyon, Professor of Sociology at Queen's University, Toronto, uses the metaphor implied by the title to examine the relationship between religion and postmodernity. Lyon's picture posits a complex set of interactions, representing an aliveness of spiritual seeking, between the stereotypical poles of the organized, complex, worldwide, media-led commercialism of Disney and the simplicity and 'unworldliness' of the originator of Christianity. Though beyond the subject of this book, its metaphor rang true with my many US experiences, especially comparing impressions from my tourist visits with sons and sister-in-law, the media picture of the country, and visits in connection with my work. The confusion I experienced in writing this chapter may therefore be a reflection of the USA as the apotheosis of postmodern contradictions. Or perhaps I didn't try hard enough.

Two promotional flyers arrived on my computer as I was preparing this final version, and they epitomize my dilemma. One for the North Carolina Council on Developmental Disabilities (2007) was for an event that promised to 'share the secrets of eight agencies that have maintained their commitment to offering only personalised supports, without exception, for one or more decades'. The other was for a new book, Dileo (2007) which, according to its pre-released foreword, demonstrates

> lack of progress due to the 'disability industrial complex' (DIC), an insidious bureaucracy of traditionalists funded by methods that serve the status quo. The DIC is based on the historical assumption that this disenfranchised group of people is best served by specialists within isolated settings, an assumption that is not only immoral but also ineffective, costly, and most certainly illegal.
>
> (Lawhead and Lawhead 2007: i)

Surface similarities between Canada and the USA – many of the same television channels, similar sports, similar size of houses and vastness of goods in the shops – are paralleled on the surface of the service system. The provision of services by agencies; the state or provincial bureaucracies administering the system; the range of agency sizes from one or two person services to multi-million dollar corporations – even the much vaunted success of inclusive education – all seem to have the same brashness, the same reliance of imagery and marketing to attract parents to use the agencies, and the same bewildering range of quality and effects on people's lives. Yet my underlying sense was of a significant contrast between the two countries.

I have already talked about the paradox of Canadian services, and perhaps it is simply that the USA is a multidimensional paradox of paradoxes, given the size of the country, the variation in levels of affluence, of political power, and of influence over both policy and practice in welfare in general, let alone intellectual disability in particular. If so, I run the risk of either describing, in Disney fashion, the 'stars of serviceland' or of being the curmudgeonly Englishman describing the appalling danger, vulgarity, bad taste, and downright decadence of the service system's reflection of its culture.

I can therefore only try, in the limited space available, to adopt the same approach to the USA as to the other countries, though with a warning as to its extra likelihood of inaccuracy and incompleteness. With those riders, that Mel Gibson (an immigrant from Australia of course) forgot to give in his interpretations of Scottish/English, American/English, and Jewish history respectively, I shall begin with an Englishman's view of US history in the field of intellectual disability.

Historical development of services

Early developments – local variation from the beginning

Early forms of 'services' in the USA are similar to other countries, often beginning some way from the large institutions and intensive eugenic programmes of the twentieth century. Wolfensberger (1970: 51) quotes Howe, for example, on his human-scale residential schools: 'organised on the family plan; the pupils all sat at the same table with the principal . . . It was the belief of managers that only a small number of inmates could be successfully cared for in our institutions.'

Even this far back, however, we get into the jungle of the US system of governance; interacting with, and part of, the national cultural values of independence and self-sufficiency, the history of slavery, dispossession and extermination of First Nations people, and discrimination against and exploitation of immigrants (Brogan 2001). The US Constitution reserves very few powers to the Federal government, with States having control over most aspects of public services. They have exercised this control in a whole range of ways, though rarely in the nineteenth century was anything like comprehensive public provision instigated, in intellectual disability or elsewhere. A contrast could possibly be made between cities and rural areas, and between the north of the country and the south (Scheerenberger 1983; Noll and Trent 2004) in terms of the development of institutions towards the end of that century, but there is no clear countrywide picture. We also need to remember that the turn of the century in the USA saw the height of the influx of the 'poor, huddled masses', that was to continue, in different forms and from different countries of origin, from then onwards, with all the resultant political and social implications. 1900 was also less than 40 years since the Civil War, with all the implications for former slaves and still remaining racial views, so again the enormity of the country, and complexity of local political issues, return.

The twentieth century – familiar and unfamiliar patterns

As the new century developed, so did industrialization and public education, with people increasingly being measured and defined as 'retarded'. As in Europe, greater recording of such assessments led to the widespread view of a 'swamping' of the nation and the fostering of eugenics. In the more practically oriented, individualistic and less class-based slant of the academic and professional sector in the USA, especially the earnestly youthful and empirical 'new sciences' of psychology, psychiatry and genetics, many studies were carried out to 'prove' the inheritability of 'retardation'. (e.g. Goddard 1912). The transatlantic exchange on this issue, including the development of the 'scientific' measure of intelligence tests, gave academic credibility to the widespread views on degeneracy, and as we have seen, personnel as well as ideas passed between the English-speaking nations, with US mobilization and testing of recruits for the 1914–18 war bringing further attention to the degree of 'retardation'. The response to these influences between the wars, still with much State variation, was the familiar building or expanding of large, segregated institutions, and the development and continued use of sterilization, both within and outside of these institutions (Trent 1994). Wolfensberger again sums it up starkly, remembering he was describing developments from the 1920s that still largely prevailed as he wrote:

> In order to segregate vast numbers of menacing deviants, institutions had to enlarge and be operated economically . . . packed like herring cans, . . . some institutions housed over 5,000 residents; expenditure was cut and economic productivity maximized. Institutions had to be built where land was the cheapest – i.e. far from centres of population. Maximized productivity specifically implied the ruthless exploitation of the labour of the resident retardate to the point of working him literally to death. Death rates in institutions were catastrophic.
>
> (Wolfensberger 1970: 52)

Post-war developments, or lack of them

Noting the lack of change since then, Wolfensberger also suggested, based on a European tour in the 1960s, that though they shared many of the same origins, there was a strong contrast in the *degree* to which the institutional regimes in the two continents affected their inmates, such that an observer of both would 'probably see less animal-like behaviour in the more severely retarded in all of Denmark or Sweden than he will in a single one of our typical American institutions' (ibid.: 52).

A further transatlantic contrast, even greater in the 1950s and 1960s, was the involvement of the *national* governments in health, education, and social services, seen before the war, not only the European countries, but even to some extent the three colonies. Federal involvement, in the USA, tended only to begin on any scale post-war (Murray 1994) and, even then did not impose policies by law or direct funding. Instead, the Federal government, then as now, designates a *constitutional basis* for action, and creates sources of funding which States can take or leave. If they accept funding, States must observe attached regulations, but otherwise plan and organize how money is spent. Over the years this has led to many disputes between State and Federal bureaucrats over interpretation, as well as huge State variation even within funding regulations. As we shall see later, this is especially important for some key sources such as Medicaid, but those sources were not in abundance in the immediate post-war period.

Normalization and community services – the 1970s and beyond

Though Wolfensberger and others from the USA were key members of the small transatlantic group involved with the development of normalization, and though his published work and the leadership group he developed were, especially through PASS and PASSING training and their offshoots, to have a worldwide effect on changing services, changes in the USA were much more haphazard, though a key similarity to other countries was the development of radical parent groups, some of whom began to campaign for alternatives to institutions, and some who set up services themselves (Menolascino et al. 1968).

The use of law, however, seems a key point of difference. In other countries we have seen either *statute law*, national or local government policies, or the lack of them, as crucial influences. In the USA, *specific law suits*, or the threat of them, also have a significant influence, and did as part of the anti-institutional movement. As usual, this is complex, with different levels of courts at both State and Federal level, as well as different *kinds* of lawsuits, especially the key distinction between *individual* cases and *class* actions, providing a maze of legal precedents and effects. The action brought on behalf of the inmates of the Willowbrook Institution in New York (Rothman and Rothman 2005) is perhaps the best-known example of a class action, and it did produce significant change in that State, but again decisions only apply to the named class on whose behalf the action is brought, and within the jurisdiction of the relevant courts.

Rizzolo et al. (2004) list ongoing legal actions affecting services in 31 different states. They note that:

> The importance of a civil rights history and a strong advocacy presence is suggested by the extent of MR/DD class action litigation in the nation after 1971 . . . This stimulated many defendant state governments to request substantial additional funds from their funding legislatures to implement new community services initiatives.
>
> (ibid.: 58)

This feature of US policy development compounds the complexity of trying to understand service history, since it went alongside the other effects we have already noted; the development of normalization, its teaching, especially via workshops; the stories from Canada of the possibility of 'comprehensive service systems'; all alongside the growth of parent groups, campaigning organisations, and the beginnings of Citizen Advocacy.

This was not all, however, and here again the variation in governance and funding play a part. We noted the gradual increase in Federal government involvement in the 1950s and 1960s, and a specific aspect of that involvement, when combined with State administrators' efforts to use it or otherwise, is another significant influence on change that continues to the present day, and one that is equally Byzantine in its operation.

Its context is various forms of welfare assistance funded or mandated by the Federal government. There have been a number of these, including a federally administered means-tested income support payment called Supplemental Security Income (SSI). For those who are eligible for SSI, services provided under the Federal funding programme known as Medicaid (MA) also apply. Similarly means tested, MA requires States who choose to use it to match Federal funds with their own, and obliges them to offer a basic set of services. States can *choose*, however, to offer a variety of other eligible services. Though MA covers such things as clinical services, hospitalizations, drugs, and nursing home services, which most people in the USA cover by private or employer-funded insurance, the key issue is *who* gets *which* MA-funded program, rather than what they get. Many people with intellectual disabilities are eligible for SSI, hence MA-funded programmes, and services have been affected significantly by the way States have used MA funding, initially via a stream called Intermediate Care Facilities for the Mentally Retarded (ICF/MR). States that chose to include this in their State Medicaid Plan received matching Federal funds according to a complex formula. 'ICF' is a generic term for a sort of nursing home for individuals assessed (by a team of professionals) as *not* requiring 'skilled nursing care'. 'ICF-MR', as the second part of the name implies, specifically relates to intellectually disabled people, but is a federally funded *programme*. *Facilities* funded by ICF-MR are not standard, but some States used the programme to provide smaller alternatives to institutions. The key appears to be how well the facilities fitted the detailed regulations and eligibility rules governing 'Intermediate Care', including issues of staffing, individual plans, monitoring, and physical setting specifications. For some States, this simply meant re-arranging things in their institutions to fit the regulations; others commissioned agencies to provide new facilities, again with a whole range of sizes. Still others tried to reduce the size of ICF-MR facilities, and succeeded in obtaining a different set of federal-approved regulations for 'ICFs-MR small' (housing 15 or fewer people). While smaller than the traditional institutions, however, such facilities tended to be just below 15, rather than well below, and still usually purpose-built, rather than ordinary housing (Taylor 2005).

So the marketplace of services began to take a broader shape, then fuelled, and made even more complex, by the introduction of the Medicaid Home and Community Based Services (HCBS) Waiver. As we have seen, both institutions and ICFs-MR could draw on MA funding. Community-based facilities other than such settings, however, had developed by the 1980s, first with group homes, then smaller places, plus more individualized services apart from residential care (Hogan 1980; O'Brien et al. 1998). Funding for these largely came from State tax revenue but then some States, with New York a leading example, sought to convert their community system to MA funding by negotiating for the Federal government to 'waive' certain of the regulations and criteria that went with existing MA-funded programmes. This was not a blanket system. Individual 'waivers' were negotiated for specific groups, and/or specific services for specific groups, all varying according to how States used MA funding, whether they saw MA waivers as a means of getting extra Federal funding, or giving them, the States, more flexibility of provision. Even within States, how services were organized more locally also contributed to demands, or the lack of them, for the State to negotiate waivers.

Rizzolo et al. chart its history as follows, confirming the still existing wide variation. 'First authorized by Congress in 1981 . . . the HCBS Waiver has now emerged as the principal Medicaid program underwriting MR/DD long-term care, surpassing Medicaid ICF/MR spending in the states in 2001' (2004: 58).

On the one hand, therefore, the history of services in the USA shows a significant change from the position in the 1960s – where, in Wolfensberger's view (1999: 56) 'Just how pessimistic and outright nihilistic people tended to be . . . and how modest the aspirations of even most advocates for the retarded were, is difficult to imagine by people who were not there at the time' – to the

1970s and 1980s, where developments gave great hopes and inspiration, not just to those in the USA but, as we have seen, elsewhere. On the other hand, the great variation in the US system, within and between States and services, combined with broader changes in funding of welfare in the USA from the Reagan government onwards, has also meant that the service system in the new millennium still has large elements of institutional provision.

Recent history has seen, to use my Disneyland analogy again, many 'stars of serviceland', who can join the parade down Main Street, but a look beneath the surface, and a look across the world beyond the stereotyped representations in the 'small world' merry-go-round, can leave immense confusion, and an underlying sense of waste, of time, money, and perhaps of lives. We shall see how this pans out in detail, after the usual summary table (Table 7.1).

Pre-natal services – the right to not exist?

> Attitudes toward congenital disability per se have not changed markedly. Both premodern as well as contemporary societies have regarded disability as undesirable and to be avoided. Not only have parents recognized the birth of a disabled child as a potentially divisive, destructive force in the family unit, but the larger society has seen disability as unfortunate . . . Our society still does not countenance the elimination of diseased/disabled people; but it does urge the termination of diseased/disabled foetuses. The urging is not explicit, but implicit.
>
> (Retsinas 1991: 91)

As we have seen from earlier chapters, Retsinas' observation of the similarity between 'our society' i.e. the USA, and others appears to have some weight. The range of practices on screening and pre-natal abortion that we have seen, however, have largely hinged on the *statutory* law on abortion, with the connection with disability being one part of a legal definition in such laws allowing abortion in specific circumstances. The 'wrongful birth' cases cited in the Australian chapter, where individuals are suing doctors, were notable because of their rarity, whereas, again, the dominance of legal action as a lead to policy still seems differentiate the USA from the other countries. What this does *not* mean, however, in my view, is a significant difference between countries in their societal attitude to disabled children that screening and selective abortion represent.

It is therefore not surprising that, in the USA, pre-natal screening for chromosomal abnormalities is routinely offered to all pregnant women who present for care by their 20th gestational week. In a survey of around 450 racially and ethnically diverse pregnant women, regarding decisions *not* to

Table 7.1 Schematic overview of 'services' that affect the lives of people with intellectual disabilities in the USA

'Service'	Formal organizational place	Specialist or generic?	Main source(s) of funding
Pre-natal services	State/local hospitals and health centres Medical practices Private hospitals and practitioners Screening clinics	Generic and specialist	State Health Departments Health Insurance
Post-natal and early childhood services	State/local hospitals and health centres Medical practices Private hospitals and practitioners Early childhood agencies, some voluntary	Generic clinical services, but agency input varying in specialization	State Developmental Disability Departments State Health Departments Health Insurance State Children and Family departments – generic Education for children 3 and over
Non-educational services for children	State provision Agencies, including those providing respite services	Specialist and generic	State Developmental Disability Departments State Health Departments Health Insurance State Children and Family departments – generic
Education services – children and young adults	Local School Boards	Generic and specialist	State Education Departments Local School Boards Federal funding for specific programs
Education services – adults	Colleges and Universities	Generic and specialist	General tertiary education funding Some from DD services
Residential services – adults	Agencies – some State direct provision Some public housing	Largely specialist	State Developmental Disability Departments State funds, State/Federal Medicaid funding or via Medicaid waivers Charitable funding

Daytime services – non-work	Agencies – some State direct provision	Largely specialist	State Developmental Disability Departments State funds, State/Federal Medicaid funding or via Medicaid waivers Charitable funding
Daytime services – work	Agencies, either supported employment or open employment or both	Largely specialist	State Developmental Disability Departments State funds, State/Federal Medicaid funding or via Medicaid waivers Charitable funding
Leisure assistance	Agencies – usually as part of broader package	Largely specialist	State Developmental Disability Departments State funds, State/Federal Medicaid funding or via Medicaid waivers Charitable funding
Advocacy services	Agencies, including parent support agencies, individual Citizen advocacy agencies, and campaigning organizations	Specialist	State funding via individual or block grants to agencies for Advocacy and Protection services Charitable funding
Financial assistance	Federal and State Social Security Income	Specialist within generic service	Federal SSI from federal funds Some states supplement from State funding
Parental 'support services'	Acting as all parents Also setting up individual or community agency	Specialist, in that all children are different	Own finances, insurance or individual funding for specific parent led initiatives

have screening, Posner et al. (2004) found some interesting differences between racial/ethnic groups, but the point for this book is the automatic offer of the tests. The degree to which such screening services offer counselling, access to termination and other health care around pregnancy then also varies, both between States, in terms of public facilities, and between public and private facilities (Asch 1999).

In my conversations with people on the 2005 visit, anecdotal support was added to the picture above, i.e. that screening is now totally common. Indeed, some insurance companies were said to put pressure on doctors to get patients to sign a form before screening tests that they will terminate if they have a 'bad result'. If a child does get to be born, however, a rather more positive picture of practice in their early life seems to emerge.

Early childhood services – early intervention, pre-school education and family support

We have already seen that differences between States over the various aspects of Medicaid have resulted in considerable variation when it comes to people with intellectual disabilities and their families. The literature and my discussions seem to agree, however, on a greater degree of consistency of practice around birth and in the early years, an impression we have seen in all the countries so far, perhaps reflecting the greater commonality of needs at that time between families in the wider population and those with a disabled child. In the USA, it may also reflect the elements of Medicaid funded programmes that are mandatory, and must be described in public state plans. They include, situations around birth, inpatient hospital, outpatient hospital, early and periodic screening, diagnosis, and treatment (commonly abbreviated to EPSDT), and some nursing facility services. How these are actually provided, in terms of direct state provision or contracting out to private or charitable providers, is what varies, but help around birth, especially what could be called medical services, seem to be consistently present. Beyond this point, too, an amendment to the Education for all Handicapped Children Act of 1975, passed by Congress in 1986, gave the same rights to 'free and appropriate' public education to *pre-school* aged children between 3 and 5, and also the option for States to establish what was called an Early Intervention Program (EIP). Most States subsequently passed their own laws to implement EIPs, usually enabling the governor to select the agency to administer the EIP, with local authorities in the counties co-ordinating specific services. A 'Service Co-ordinator' is usually appointed to qualifying families, also helping them access the mandatory programmes mentioned above, though eligibility for one does not automatically guarantee eligibility for the other.

The material regarding, and observation of, the EIP in New York state that I encountered on my visit appeared impressive. More so when taken with other forms of community-based family support, in and beyond the early years, administered or financed by State MR/DD agencies, such as vouchers, direct cash payments to families, reimbursement, or direct payments to service providers which the state agencies identify as family support (New York State, undated). As with all services in the USA, however, the *entitlement*, and the possibility of lawsuits around it, take up much space in the various guides to early intervention and other family support programmes, with the onus on families to apply for support, and to pursue the application through appeals processes if necessary. In addition, there appears to be significant variation between States in terms of their use of cash payments or vouchers, where the onus is again on the parents to then go out and find services on which to spend such financial benefits, as opposed to the offer of services to meet family support needs. Where direct services are offered, there is again a range of provision, including the situation where such services are dominated by 'out of home' respite care in a range of facilities, including institutions. Rizzolo et al. (2004) do not give detailed explanations for the differential spending by States on community-based support services they present, but my conversations suggested a combination of two key reasons. First, key differences in the level of take-up in the various States, especially between poor families and others and linked to the amount of publicity given to the availability of services. Second, tensions between economies of *co-ordination*, realized by simply giving out vouchers and cash, and economies of *cost* through the provision or funding of institutional care. The latter is discussed by Rosenau (2000) in a review of what she calls 'permanency planning' for children with intellectual disabilities, i.e. the fulfilment of the expressed desire in the rhetoric of policy for children to grow up in families. Noting a net increase in admissions and readmissions to out of home residential services for children, including those under 3, in the latest available year of her study, 1998, she concludes that 'the family support movement must embrace more fully the issue of permanency' (ibid.: 3). As elsewhere, even data between States do not fully deal with the variability at local level, and here we return to the complexity of the USA. The broader data that I have used do not provide information at this level, and therefore I am more reliant on discussions that suggest the importance of really local commitment. States that delegate down to county or even lower level administration of systems can aid this process, though one does not necessarily follow the other. Where there is a major issue locally to help a child to remain in their home, then the mobilization of both formal and informal supports seems to have occurred in a number of instances (O'Brien, pers. comm. 2006). As a positive corollary to the notion, valued in the USA, of independent communities 'looking after their own' such local efforts challenge my Disneyland analogy, at least in terms of its critique of Disney's over-reliance on imagery rather than substance, and is a key issue for this chapter, well beyond childhood services.

Moving on to pre-school provision, we have already noted the mandatory nature of access to pre-school educational services, provided families apply and are deemed to be eligible. We can use the guidelines for pre-school education in New York State (New York State Education Department 2002) as an example, and I was told, and observed from examination of some others, that, in *procedures* at least, there is a more consistency across States. These guidelines form part of broader guidelines covering school education as a whole, and considerable space is allocated to rights of appeal, legal boundaries of provision, and distinctions between pre-school and school-aged children. A child has to be allocated to a category of disability that falls within the range of categories defined by the Commissioner of Education via its local Committees on Pre-School Special Education (CPSEs), which are set up in each school district in any particular state. For a school-aged child, categories tend to be those of Federal law.

Reading the New York definitions, only the most obvious cases of intellectual disability, such as Down's syndrome, or people with multiple disabilities, seem to be represented in the pre-school categories. Children from poor families, the main source of students with 'learning disabilities', 'emotional disturbance', and 'mild mental retardation', (Reschly 1997; Patton 1998) which categories are added at school age, would therefore be less likely to be able to take advantage of free pre-school programmes, if the classifying regime were strict. Equally, as I found in my discussions with Jowonio, pre-school programmes such as theirs, which is in the private sector, do not automatically fall under the provision offered by New York State, even if children are deemed eligible, since the State will look first at its public schooling provision.

Each school district, the local administrative area for public education with its own elected board, employed bureaucracy, and considerable autonomy, will have a Committee on Special Education (with a variety of names) with either a sub-committee or separate group to deal with pre-school services. If a child is deemed eligible, either at pre-school or school age, then there is an obligation for these committees to draw up an Individualized Education Plan (IEP). In many States, parents are said to be 'part of' the CSEs, when it comes to drawing up the plan, but there is also provision, as usual for those who can afford it, for an independent appraisal of the child. If the IEP is drawn up at pre-school level, there still needs to be a referral to the main CSE as the child comes up to school age. This is done, in the words of the guidelines, if the CPSE decides that 'your child continues to have a disability and/or if he or she continues to require special education programs or services. If so, the CPSE will make a referral to the CSE' (New York State guidelines 2002: 9).

So, as Adam's World Tour box reveals, if he were conceived in the USA, and got to be born, there would be much he, and we his parents, would be *entitled* to, by way of rights to services in his early childhood – what we would get would depend a lot on who, and where we were.

ADAM'S WORLD TOUR

Conceived in the USA – what next?

The pressures from insurance and our 'rights' to a trouble-free birth and child free from disability, combined with the ready availability of abortion, would be set against the part of the USA in which we were, and what our economic status was, in determining Adam's likelihood of being born. In a number of States, counter-pressures from anti-abortion groups could affect the availability of, or our access to, clinics, especially if we were poor, though an average standard of living, especially with health insurance, would mean we were pretty much free to respond to the inevitable offer of screening and its results.

If Adam were born, then again who we were, and where we lived, would be important, though as a person with an obvious intellectual disability like Down's syndrome, perhaps less so in Adam's early years. How our State's legislature acted in light of its interest in making the most of federal funding and how our State's executive has planned, including its negotiations with federal authorities around jointly funded programmes and other support around Adam's birth would be one factor. Then how it interpreted the pre-school educational legislation, though there would be a 'right' to at least some support. Whether some of this support was 'out of home' and where that might be in terms of a facility, would also be affected by the State, not just by whether they chose to give support in terms of cash or vouchers, as opposed to direct services, but also the sort of direct services they had on offer. It would normally be our responsibility to apply for support of both kinds, since though there are mandated outreach efforts their effectiveness seems quite variable, and for the pre-school education we would need to go through the school district committees to determine eligibility and then an IEP. If Adam had not had an IEP by the time he came up to school age, he would definitely get one then, as a child with Down's syndrome, though if he had less obvious intellectual disabilities, especially if we were poor and relatively inarticulate, a classification as disabled might not come until later. On the other hand, it appears that poor children tend to be over-diagnosed, especially if they are black or Hispanic boys. This would also depend, not just on the State's interpretation of the legislation, but the practices of the school district in which we lived. Again, if we were of average income or above, other options than those provided or funded by the state would be available, including those, like Jowonio, that espoused a particular educational philosophy, and even then they can offer some degree of flexibility in fee levels in line with certain philosophies.

Education – inclusion rights, and inclusion realities

The above title has deliberately been repeated from the preceding chapter as an indication that many issues around education, perhaps more so than in other services, appear to be similar between the USA and Canada. The similarity appears to come in the intangible process by which the notion of inclusion has achieved a degree of acceptance in the two countries. We have seen how the welfare states of Scandinavia determined centrally that there would be inclusion, and how the total dominance of public provision in education means that the central policy can be put into practice. On the other hand, national or regional policy within systems, allowing significant overt or covert selection by price, geographical location or professional fiefdoms, as in New Zealand, Australia, and as we shall see, the UK, has meant inclusion has been less fully accepted or implemented. Canada and the USA seem closer in their education systems to this latter group of countries, yet the degree of inclusion appears to be greater. Not comprehensive, however, as illustrated by the other similarity between the two North American countries, that despite the achievement of legal 'rights' to inclusion, children are still excluded, as we noted in the quotation from Michael Bach at the beginning of the Canada chapter.

Certainly, as that chapter discussed, normalization radicals of the early 1970s found ready allies in the education field, with many in fact coming from that field. This provided fertile ground for the development of the sorts of innovative project that was Jowonio school in its early days and is now represented by work such as Biklen et al. (2003). The McGill summer schools of the 1980s and 1990s in Montreal were attended by many teachers and administrators from both sides of the border, attempting to respond to the inclusive legislation of the 1970s and 1980s in a positive fashion, and developing a number of North American networks which often overlapped a normalization background and a radical education approach. It would therefore be possible for one of those networks, in its later manifestation as the University of Kansas Circle of Inclusion (http://circleofinclusion.org/) to be able to quote hard evidence of the success of inclusion in both popular newsletter pronouncements and academic publications. More important still, almost two generations of teachers in training received the inclusion message, and it seems to have been the professional acceptance of at least a critical mass of teachers in North America that has led to the successes of inclusion (Biklen et al. 2003).

Federal and State initiatives have also helped, though given the structure of school governance in the USA, with the responsibility for education resting with locally elected school boards and much educational provision financed by local taxes (typically local property taxes), their initiatives are more incentives than mandates. At Federal level, there have been various education laws, beginning with the Education for All Handicapped Children Act 1975 up to the No Child left Behind Act of 2001 and the more recent Individuals with Disabilities Education Improvement Act of 2004 that have attempted, with some success, to ensure the rights of all children to attend publicly funded schooling alongside their peers. This is done, however, through the medium of Federal funding, still a small part of overall school funding, having strings attached in terms of 'measurements of progress' which are open to degrees of interpretation.

On the extent of inclusion, we can possibly judge further from the National Longitudinal Transition Study (NLTS) (http://www.sri.com/policy/cehs/publications/dispub/nlts/nltssum.html), originally conducted 1987–93, then followed up in the new millennium. Their main study data (implying 83 per cent attendance of intellectually disabled children in mainstream schools) can certainly be used to support a notion that inclusion of children with disabilities has 'happened', and the later follow-up studies maintain the overall trend (NCSER 2006), and *also* found, however, that those in the 'mental retardation' and 'multiple disability' categories had the lowest numbers, at 44.4 per cent and 31.7 per cent respectively, actually *in mainstream classrooms*. Some 27.8 per cent and 54.6 per cent of these students spent less than a quarter of their *time* in mainstream classrooms, despite being 'included' in the school.

The age-related degree of inclusion in the USA seems to have greater similarity with elsewhere. In the early years, opportunities for and practice of inclusion seem to be fairly high, borne out by my discussions with Jowonio, among others. After pre-school, the tendency is also that the CSE process means children go to their local school. Some pre-school educational services, including inclusive schools like Jowonio, do a lot of work with mainstream schools before people go, and in an area like Syracuse, with its long history of commitment to inclusion, its closeness and attachment to the university via student placements, training events, etc., a significant 'culture of inclusion' can build up. Once children are deemed eligible for special education, their IEP must be reviewed every three years, and again there appears to be more focus on this in the initial school years. When children get to the 'middle school' years (defined differently in different states, but roughly 10–13 years of age), the ability to achieve real inclusion seems to be affected by more schools creating segregated units, or, conversely, claiming that they cannot provide 'a suitable environment' because they do not have units. Children can then get channelled to schools which do have these facilities.

The entitlement that goes with a State's acceptance of Federal education funds is to a 'free and appropriate public education' as determined by the IEP process. If what is deemed appropriate is only provided in a few places in a State, because of the 'economic' sharing of schools for 'low incidence populations' (usually severely disabled children) among school districts, then this may mean bussing them for hours. It may well be cheaper for States to fund the contract with the bus company than to set up more such schools, or persuade the mainstream schools to include whatever particular 'special educational need' the schools or programmes claim to meet. This can also, I was told, lead to parents trying to persuade the State that particular 'special schools', are the only places where their child's needs can be met. Similarly, at high school level, what is offered to parents from the mainstream can lead them to opt for special schools as the alternative.

Yet again, therefore, in fact more so in the US culture, the key role of parents/supporters in getting more radical things for their children emerges, but also the 'blinkers' of some States and School Boards, despite clear evidence of more radical things working (Bunch and Valeo 1997). The wide variation in practice, across and within States, as people go through the school system, seems, ironically, to give narrower options as the end of school approaches. Like Canada, American young people with disabilities can stay on at high school until they are 21, with a strong emphasis on vocational, rather than academic, programmes being provided. NTDS figures again put this into context. They report, from their later survey, that 'relatively few' 15–19-year-olds in the 'mentally retarded' and 'multiply disabled' categories are out of school (19 per cent and 14 per cent, respectively), and note that these figures are consistent with those from the U.S. Department of Education (2003) in revealing the tendency of these groups to remain in high school until they reach age 21. NDTS also note that young people in the above categories who *have* left high school 'are among the least likely to have completed high school (72 per cent and 65 per cent), and within the group of completers, they are among the least likely to be reported by parents to have graduated with a regular diploma (84 per cent and 91 per cent)' (NCSER 2006: 13).

As we move on to consider what happens to people after they have left school, therefore, Adam's World Tour box reinforces the issues of location and parental effort and income, in determining what his experiences at school in the USA might be.

ADAM'S WORLD TOUR

Going to school in the USA

As parents, we have a lot of 'rights' to educational services for Adam. What we will actually get seems to depend a lot on whether we exercise those rights, which in turn depends on which State and community we are in, whether we are in a rural or urban part of it, and our income and ability to articulate our claims. Adam's rights to, and granting of eligibility for, pre-school programmes and then his entry into the school system would also be affected by those factors, but for as obvious a condition as Down's syndrome, it is likely we would have had an IEP in place before Adam came up to school age, and possibly an inclusive pre-school place. It is also likely that our School District, especially if we were in an urban area, would place Adam in our local mainstream school, if that is what we wanted. If we wanted special schooling, or a school with a particular 'special programme', then how much we could choose in the marketplace would depend on the IEP interpretation of what was 'appropriate', on referral and money from School Districts, or possibly if we had a high level of income. Depending on the local policy of shared facilities between School Districts, and Adam's IEP, we might see Adam bussed to a school or programme some way across the State. If we left it to the system, then the degree of full inclusion of Adam would depend on the age level of the school, with more happening at elementary level, less at middle school, and less still at high school, depending on State and School District belief that the IEP objectives could be achieved in an integrated setting – a fairly frequent occurrence, I was told.

As Adam went through middle and high school, probably staying until he was 20/21, his curriculum would tend to be more vocationally oriented, and he would be likely to be less often with his age peers in the regular classroom. He would also have a relatively low chance of 'graduating' fully from high school, though 'modified graduation' might well be given. As for transition to post-school, he would almost always be referred to the state 'Department of Mental Retardation' (under a variety of names).

Throughout the whole process, if we had sufficient income and energy, then legal action to ensure our 'rights', to appeal against local CSE decisions, or simply to move to a State that fitted our wishes for Adam, would all be possibilities. This would seem to be the case for a majority, though not an overwhelming one, of parents in the USA, and is anticipated in the amount of space given to the eligibility and appeals processes within the overall system. This facet of services would continue as Adam left school.

Daytime services – workshops, community activities and real work

All the countries described so far have competitive industrialized economies, with increasing demands for intellectual and social skills, as opposed to manual labour, and unionization of labour, if varying in degree (KILM 2005). One offshoot of this state of affairs is the impression that no country could be said to have 'cracked' the issue of open, paid employment for people with intellectual disabilities. The thinking necessary for employers to believe that it is worth hiring a person with a disability, especially an intellectual disability, is still somewhat radical. With as strong legislation as most, and also with probably the widest range of levels of employment possibilities and weakest overall union power (Chaison 2005), the USA should be in a position to lead the way in open employment. Overviews of the situation in practice could make a case that it does so, with a proportion of some 24 per cent of people in all US 'day programs' designated by Rizzolo et al. (2004: 27–8) as being in 'supported or competitive employment'. Their figures show considerable growth in numbers in this category from 1988–93, slowing in the next ten years, and with the growth in spending also slowing from 2000–2. They also show a considerable range across States, with four having a proportion of less than 10 per cent, while eight States have 40 per cent or more.

Two issues therefore re-appear: what is defined as 'work', for people with intellectual disabilities; and the large variation between both the US States' expenditures and the different kinds of services they provide (Gilmore and Butterworth 1997; Cohen et al. 2003; Larson et al. 2004), with the familiar issue that most of the Federal legal and/or financial initiatives for daytime activities in relation to work, though substantial, have been optional. Along with those initiatives reflected in the growth rates cited above by Rizzolo et al. (2004) have often come specific efforts regarding transition, but, as we saw earlier, of all the disability groups, transition from school seemed to take place later for young people with intellectual disabilities. Most young people with clearly identified intellectual disabilities, such as Down's syndrome, remain at school until they are 21 and then, if they have not already been, are referred to the State Department of Mental Retardation (DMR hereafter, though actually going under a variety of names in different States). How commissioning, covering services in *all* aspects of people's lives, is then administered varies by State, with some managing most things from State level, while others allow considerable autonomy at lower levels of local government. This then also affects how they use the various funding sources, especially the Medicaid waiver options, to purchase from agencies, though many States are also direct providers of services.

Most States also use MA funding for workers involved with the service allocation process, mostly organized in parallel with the delegation or otherwise of local commissioning. These people, most commonly called 'service co-ordinators' are normally the access point to the DMR system, though parents often choose to find agencies that suit them, usually with help from local advisory groups. Further complications come with States, or lower levels of administration, assigning responsibility for *commissioning* to agencies, sometimes agencies that also provide services. Nor is there usually an organizational distinction between commissioners of day and residential services. Advice given to parents, and what might be offered to them, therefore comes from a variety of sources, with a variety of interests, even assuming they get past the basic DMR eligibility process. DMR caseworkers will inevitably have pressures to fit State priorities, whether those are budgetary, to reduce waiting lists, and/or to comply with the results of court judgements (usually for those certified as members of a class on whose behalf an action was brought). If advisors are from agencies, they may have a vested interest in promoting their agency's services, especially some of the very large agencies, some of which have grown from parents' organizations. Other agencies not involved in direct provision, ironically sometimes local offshoots of national parents' organizations, or sometimes organizations such as Citizen Advocacy offices, will give possibly different advice. Most States specify that people should have an 'annual plan', but this too can be the source of a whole range of such documents, from a simple note of 'more of the same' to elaborate variations on the theme of 'person centred approaches' (O'Brien et al., 1997).

A key issue in recent years has been the development of 'individualized funding', noted in other countries earlier in the book. In 2002, a study was carried out for the National Association of State Directors of Developmental Disabilities Services (NASDDDS) (Moseley et al. 2003) on the amount and processes of 'individualized funding initiatives', i.e. those where money is specifically allocated to individuals to work out and pay for some sort of organized support, as opposed to slotting them into existing funded services. Some 43 of the 51 State Intellectual Disabilities Departments responded to the survey, with individual budgeting options being available in 75 per cent of them, though even here described as the 'exception rather than the rule'.

So as well as the locality you live in determining the *people you will have to deal with* to get services, it will also determine whether services will be offered from direct State provision or the buying of agency services, whether there will be an individualized allocation process, and whether particular groups or particular services can be funded this way. The NASDDDS survey (Moseley et al. 2003) found a number of key variants between States; by funding source, service category, provider type, and administering authority; by the process for determining an 'Allocation Amount'; whether there was a spending limit on such programmes; and the variation in involvement of families and advocates in the process, and thus how much of a negotiation, as opposed to a simple allocation of a budget, takes place.

Also, whatever is done on the 'daytime' end of things will often be part of a total package involving other aspects of life. Clearly, in those states that have a high percentage of institutional places, there would be a greater probability that people in institutions spend a good part of their day there. Even people living with parents or relatives, however, can be directed towards 'respite', in various forms of segregated provision, during the daytime, as well as what is called a 'day program'. Probably the majority, again supported by survey data, (Rizzolo et al. 2004) would be people in segregated sheltered workshops, day programs called 'community involvement' or 'individualized day programs' which were often, more cruelly, called 'mall therapy' by critics.

'Empty days', of course, is a situation that could be found in most of the countries of this book, especially those whose service provision is based to a significant extent on independent agencies, but the degree of grouping together of a disparate range of service users is perhaps more specific to US services. As we have seen, given the basis of funding and allocation of services to adults with intellectual disabilities, such a complex picture was repeated when it came to residential services.

Residential services – beyond group homes to 'welcoming communities?'

> The shift to self-directed services and the implementation of individual budgeting methodologies requires states to change many of the fundamental policies and practices that have sustained developmental disabilities systems over the years. The results of this study also suggest that a successful transition cannot be achieved through incremental adjustments in the status quo, but rather require focused attention to fundamentally alter all aspects of program delivery.
>
> (Moseley et al. 2003: 21)

Moseley et al.'s conclusions highlight, for me, both the possibilities and difficulties of achieving the sort of lives for people that a number in the USA have reached, and which match the best of any of the countries I have visited (O'Brien et al. 1998; Carlson 2000). As we have already seen in relation to daytime activity, the possibilities are found in the freedom provided by the system of agency funding and devolution to local stakeholders, especially in the form of individualized budgets. The difficulties seem to occur when that same freedom is used by States to look for simple solutions that minimize cost, and/or adopt what John O'Brien (2005) calls the 'path of compliance', i.e. doing the minimum that is required by law, or the regulations of funding streams. Even what has been hailed as a 'landmark case', which forms the precedent for the great majority of current court actions (Rizzolo et al. 2004) the so-called 'Olmstead case' (*Olmstead v L.C* 1999) has been responded to in a variety of ways. This Supreme Court judgment called for residential and other services to be provided, which 'enable individuals with disabilities to interact with non-disabled individuals to the fullest extent possible'. This could, and has been, used to bolster reform efforts such as those in Wisconsin (O'Brien and O'Brien 2006). The fact that so many actions are still outstanding, however, and so many people are still in institutional settings, highlights the difficulties of such reforms within current systems, especially when faced with budgetary cutbacks that have come with the Bush administration nationally and its dealings with the States and localities, so graphically illustrated by the hurricane Katrina episode.

Even where legal action is successful, the fundamental reform of a system which allows States to maintain large institutions seems far from being achieved. A case from 2004 in California perhaps illustrates the point. After two years of their suit, Davis et al. (v. California Health and Human Services Agency et al. 2004) successfully challenged the practice of the city of San Francisco, in serving people with disabilities in the Laguna Honda Hospital and Rehabilitation Center (LHH), a 1,200-bed nursing home. The judgment required San Francisco to develop a system of assessment and hospital-discharge planning that allowed people in LHH, or eligible for admission, the *option* of receiving supports and services in the community. As well as developing this 'new' system, the city had to agree to provide *training* on 'community-living alternatives' for staff and 'training and support resources' for LHH residents. The case had challenged the State Mental Health Department's Pre-Admission Screening and Resident Review programme, which it was claimed 'steered' people towards institutional care, and the plaintiffs were assisted by a 'friend of the court brief' from the US Department of Justice (DOJ). The DOJ also questioned the cost-effectiveness of San Francisco's plan to spend $401 million for a 1,200-bed replacement facility that would have cost $127,000 per bed each year to operate, noting that 'community integrated options could be provided at a fraction of the cost of staying in LHH'. On the face of it, this is a 'success' for those wanting community alternatives, but to the outsider such as myself, along with other data from surveys of provision, evaluations, and personal experiences from those I met on my visit, there are more worrying aspects, especially that it took a court case to get San Francisco to react to the Olmstead judgment, rather than the evidence of many years of work on community options. We have noted that developments in the US system do tend to be influenced by court judgments, but with so many published accounts of successful community integration, one might have thought that States would have moved in that direction without waiting to be sued.

Instead, it would not have been, one suspects, unique across the USA that the city of San Francisco was planning the 1,200-bed replacement facility, nor that the headline around the Davis case in 2004 was 'California Settlement Takes *First Step* Toward Olmstead Compliance' (my emphasis).

A further concern from the California example is that, like the *Olmstead* case, and the policy process it represents, it can be read as reinforcing the notion of a spectrum of care that is associated with a spectrum of people. Taylor (2005) points to a range of historical uses of phrases like 'least restrictive', 'most integrated', 'most normalising', and so on, not neccessarily being all to do with pioneering moves, and leading to a misconceived concept of a 'continuum' of services, especially residential, through which people pass until they reach their 'proper level'. Apart from this sometimes simply renaming the status quo, Taylor also points out that the continuum concept embeds degrees of segregation and specific physical settings as an inevitable response to this continuum. Hence his chapter title, 'The Institutions are Dying, but Are Not Dead Yet'. Thus the San Francisco judgment points to people being given the *option* of community services or the institution, with the implication that people would either choose or need to stay in the latter, or its $401 million replacement. John O'Brien's (2005) reflections on approaches in response to *Olmstead* concur with Taylor's refutation of the notion of parallel spectrums of people and services, and his and others' work provide powerful evidence of the possibility of people of whatever level of impairment leading fulfilling lives in communities (O'Brien et al. 2003; Allen et al. 2005).

These concerns seem to be supported by statistical surveys, which while limited as to the actual *quality* of the various environments, at least give a picture of the huge variety of residential care practices in the various States of the USA. In their major research brief of the developments following the introduction of the 'Medicaid waiver', Lakin and Prouty (2003) confirm the overall move during the 20 years from the original Budget Reconciliation Act of 1981 towards the use of waivers to fund community-based alternatives to institutional care, which we noted in the historical section above.

> States differ greatly in their overall use of HCBS, their rate of expansion of HCBS over the past decade, and in their relative commitment to HCBS as an alternative to ICF-MR. . . . Medicaid HCBS programs have grown at remarkable rate in the first two decades of since their authorization, and especially in the most recent decade. They have truly transformed the focus of Medicaid long-term care supports for persons with ID/DD from an overwhelmingly institutional service program to a predominantly community service program. HCBS growth, the changing demand and expectations for services, and the socio-economic realities facing the nation and individual states will all contribute to notable challenges to future development and maintenance of HCBS programs.
>
> (ibid.: 2–4)

The variation between States and its application to the broader residential care picture is confirmed by later figures from Prouty et al. (2006), showing the following

- In 2005, 41 States were operating at least one large state facility.
- The reduction in size of residential facilities, however, has led to the overall *number* of settings 'growing very rapidly'.

- Some 98 per cent of residential facilities were provided by 'non-state' agencies, who also had a very high proportion of 'small' residences (98.5 per cent of all settings with 15 or fewer residents, and 98.9 per cent of the settings with 6 or fewer, as opposed to 78.9 per cent of facilities with 16 or more residents).

- In terms of numbers of *people*, as opposed to facilities, about 83.7 per cent of those receiving residential services lived in places with 15 or fewer residents, 70.8 per cent with 6 or fewer residents, and 44.8 per cent with 3 or fewer residents. A substantial majority of people receiving residential services from non-state agencies lived in smaller settings, while a substantial majority who lived in state residences lived in large facilities.

- Interstate variability was again confirmed, with one State (Mississippi) reporting a *majority* of people in facilities of 16 or more residents, though the national average was 16.3 per cent. In 46 States, the majority received residential services in settings with *6 or fewer* residents. Among the 42 States for which such data were available, people living in settings of *3 or fewer* residents ranged from 0.0 per cent to 94.3 per cent of all those receiving residential services.

- Regardless of size, two-thirds of people receiving residential services lived in what the authors defined as 'congregate care settings', being those where 'care is provided in settings owned, rented or managed by the residential services provider, or the provider's agents in which paid staff come to the settings to provide care, supervision, instruction and other support'. The remaining third of the residential service population is made up of 25 per cent of people in their 'own home' which they own or rent, and about 8 per cent in host family/foster care. Both of these latter categories are reported as growing, but slowly, again with large State variation

- 'Own home' should be distinguished from the 'family home', i.e. with parents or other relatives. An estimated 56.5 per cent of all persons receiving services lived in family homes.

- Finally, the survey estimated that there were nearly 74,000 persons waiting for residential services (just under half the number actually receiving them). To remove that waiting list would require an estimated overall 18 per cent growth in available residential service capacity, but with huge State variation, ranging from zero growth to 173.6 per cent.

The picture, therefore, of residential services is very mixed, though it reflects all that has gone before, and, as we have noted, obviously has an impact on both daytime activities and the situation of families whose disabled member is on the waiting list. This brings us back to the role played by parents and advocates of people in developing the movements within services that represent the top end of the spectrum – indeed, in challenging the notion of a spectrum at all.

Parents, advocates and supporters – citizenship or community membership?

In the previous chapter we saw how one of the key forces involved in the development of normalization, including the involvement of Wolfensberger and his cadre of leaders, were parent groups in Canada and the USA. The impact of the ENCOR project in Nebraska (Schalock 2002) was certainly felt in the UK in the 1970s when I was involved with the first group home, and here again, the role of the parents group in Eastern Nebraska was significant. We also talked about Wolfensberger's analysis of the various stages of voluntary organizations, and speculated on whether Canadian ACLs were at the second, service-providing, stage, or had moved on to the third, campaigning and advocating, stage. The mixed bag we saw in Canada is repeated in spades in the USA, with the additional problem of State variation affecting the form of parental and other campaigning and its targets. In addition, as we have repeated often, the route of legal action is much more common and the beneficiaries of actions, the 'classes' identified (and their parents) may have a very different experience than those at home waiting for results. Similarly, parents whose offspring pass the professionally determined criteria for certain sorts of care (especially those institutions deemed to 'need' high levels and ranges of such professionals) will draw on many more dollars than those who keep people in the family home despite varying levels of support. It is no surprise that the roots of, and still probably the greatest number of examples of, Citizen Advocacy, are found in the USA. To people in England, and more so in Scandinavia, the notion of citizen action, including collective parental action, is tempered by trust in the welfare state and professionalism, only latterly being channelled into 'issue groups', whereas in the USA it appears to be a way of life. This must be tempered, however, by reflections from events following the Katrina disaster. The assumption of taking action, often through the courts, sits for me very much alongside the notion of individual responsibility that underpins the funding of welfare and health care in the USA. This seems to be based on the idea that it is up to the individual citizen to make provision for themselves and their families, and that too much provided by the State, even via national insurance, or even shared collectively with similar groups, undermines that responsibility:

> In the rest of the industrialized world, it is assumed that the more equally and widely the burdens of illness are shared, the better off the population as a whole is likely to be. The reason the United States has forty-five million people without coverage is that its health-care

> policy is in the hands of people who disagree, and who regard health insurance not as the solution but as the problem.
>
> (Gladwell 2005: 7)

My point is not just about the inequity of US health care, but the underlying assumption that people will only be motivated to use health care that they pay for if they *really* need it, and that this is reflected in a number of States' attitude to intellectual disability services. They seem to hold the view that if community-based services are what parents and advocates *really feel people need*, then they will form action groups, go to court, and so on. The fact that such groups and people with intellectual disabilities themselves *have* taken action in a number of places, and that some really progressive things have happened, is not, it appears, sufficient for a number of States to take full action in response, especially as they also have evidence that there are plenty of parents prepared to let them get on with providing or commissioning services in their own way. Indeed, some parent groups and organizations have a major vested interest in the status quo. Even where there are a higher proportion of parents and advocates taking action than elsewhere, the size of the service system appears to be able to channel that action into individualized pockets, indeed using those pockets often to demonstrate their progressiveness, as in the Disneyland 'star parade'. On the other hand, the literature on those projects (O'Brien et al. 2003) points most frequently to the efforts of small communities coming together as a key to their success, thus making even State-wide change an unlikely phenomenon.

So there is a paradox for me at the heart of the US system, which is reflected in the Adam's World Tour box. This is that the possibility of, and knowledge of, many radical things for people with intellectual disabilities exists, but that receiving these not only depends on which State you are in, but which *local community* you are part of. Also therefore, whether you have the resources to move and/or the energy and support to develop the community where you are, including the readiness to create your own services. From comments from my visit, parents in the USA vary more than most in terms of support for radical things. Where collective organization and/or training (such as the Partners in Policymaking course, (http://www. partnersinpolicymaking.com/) or the leadership programmes run by Debbie Reidy (http://www.reidyassociates.org/index.html) in some parts of the USA) has taken place, they seem powerful in using the system to demand change – where not, not. The same goes for self-advocates. Once again, the USA seems the natural home for such a notion, with its individualistic basis, and once again there are some prime examples of highly successful individuals and groups. The system is there for the using, though as usual there is the tendency for the more articulate disabled people, not as frequently those with intellectual disabilities, to dominate, with some dangers in terms of the more vulnerable missing out.

ADAM'S WORLD TOUR

An adult citizen of the USA

If Adam had been to a mainstream school, he would probably have been involved with vocational programmes, but would also have been encouraged to stay on at school until he was 20 or 21. Depending significantly on which State we were living in, or even which part of the State, our access to whatever their Department of Mental Retardation (whatever it was called) would take a number of forms. We may even have already been receiving some financial or respite services and the school will normally have set up a Transition Plan, whose annual reviews would include service co-ordinators from the DMR, at whatever level they organized or delegated service commissioning. Of course, if he were already in residential care as a child (not as frequently occurring as before, but still probably more often than most of the other countries), Adam could well pass on to the adult system in the same institution. Much more likely is that, once Adam left school, we would be offered either a place in a sheltered workshop, or a combination of this and 'community activities'. If we wished Adam to go into a job, then sheltered work in a real work environment, or full open employment, could also be a possibility, again depending on our local community, how it used the opportunities for such programmes, how the State supported them, the availability of agencies who provided them, and whether they had vacancies. If we wished Adam to move out from the family home (or he did), that would again depend on the State, on how active we were as parents, and what advocacy or other support systems were around in our area. Those factors would also affect Adam's chances of receiving individualized funding, since States vary as to whether they use this form of funding, and for what sorts of service. If Adam could be part of a class action, perhaps following *Olmstead*, our chances of getting what we wanted might be better, though the funding of court action, unless we had funds as parents, would again depend on the nature of our community, possible support agencies, and the availability of *pro bono* lawyers or legal campaigning groups. In fact, the first two of those factors might well affect whether we even thought about Adam's life in terms of 'services' as opposed to the supports necessary for him to lead an 'ordinary life'. If we did still think in terms of services, we would need to be aware of our State's waiting lists for those services, as some States have waiting lists bigger than the current number of people receiving services, especially in residential care. On the other hand, if we behaved in the archetypical American way of self-help, citizen action, and assertion of rights, we might get a life for Adam which, paradoxically, would enable *him* to have the range of choices and relationships enjoyed by a few, but a significant few, people with intellectual disabilities in the USA. This would be more difficult if we were poor, however, almost regardless of Adam's level of disability, and even of our particular community. We would also be more likely to see Adam in a nursing home as he got older, less so if we were in a State, or part of one, that had taken the *Olmstead* case as an opportunity to develop individualized services, but then if we were in such a community, many more things would probably have happened well before Adam reached old age.

In the end we are back to Disneyland, with the impressive parade of things of wonder assumed to give satisfaction by simply being there. The wonders of some US services, I believe, disguise (through no fault of their own) the underlying forces that make their achievement even more special, but also suspend the reality of life at home for the spectators – the ordinary family and person with an intellectual disability – which is far from wonderful.

England
Home and beauty?

So she sat on with closed eyes, and half believed herself in Wonderland, though she knew she had but to open them again, and all would change to dull reality.

(Lewis Carroll)

Introduction

This chapter will differ in some ways from those that have gone before. First, there will be no 'Instant Impacts box' since, though not dull, the reality of home did not lend itself to such thoughts, more a gradual reflection as I began the process of writing. I will also be describing England, rather than Great Britain or the United Kingdom. It would certainly be possible to write about services in the larger groupings, but the subtleties of and current rapid changes in the devolution of powers to the constituent countries would use too much space in explanation compared to the actual difference in services. In addition, this chapter contrasts Adam's actual experiences with answers I would give to my questions when overseas, so such answers should be about the country in which Adam lives, and in which he had the real experiences.

England is home, the country that enabled my sister-in-law Jenny to become a citizen and paid worker in the 1970s, when very few people with Down's syndrome, or their families, would ever have dreamed such a thing were possible. It is where, 20 years later, a young man with Down's syndrome attended regular school, attained grades in public examinations greater than some of his non-disabled contemporaries, got himself a job, and was looking to move out of the family home. To this observer, it appears that he did all this while being born in a period that, despite major changes in the nature of both English society and its services for people with intellectual disabilities, still did not make such achievements commonplace. This provides the context for the 'home' chapter.

Historical development of services

Initial factors – a history of class

Earlier chapters have discussed the situation of people with intellectual disabilities in the first half of the twentieth century, with particular additions for the various countries, especially how they adopted eugenic policies. What I would add for this English chapter, though it, too, has been hinted at, is the combination of the above with the immensely powerful and deep-rooted class system of this country.

Trying to explain the subtleties of this system, the way in which it creeps into the unconscious of most people, and how it is reinforced in subtle and more crass ways by the English media, in particular, the tabloid press, I found as difficult on my trip as explaining cricket to all but the Antipodeans. But I cannot emphasize enough the part class plays in English society, not least in the relative valuations of social roles, and though its power is often attributed, at a superficial level, to the Victorian period, most serious commentators agree that it has much older origins (Thompson 1991). Key among these would be the eleventh-century Norman invasion that effectively established the aristocracy of England; successive power struggles between elements of that aristocracy in the next five hundred years; its relationship with the rise of Protestantism and the peculiar local version of that in the establishment of the Church of England; the brief but important period of Parliamentary rule in the seventeenth century, and the typically British compromise of the 'glorious revolution' of 1688, effectively creating power for a Parliament of 'commons' (who were far from common, being essentially landowners and their placemen) but without reducing the status (and wealth) of the monarchy and aristocracy, or the hereditary principle that has seen German monarchs and their descendants on the throne of England since 1714.

While the rest of Europe resounded to the effects of the French Revolution and religious wars in the late eighteenth and early nineteenth centuries, England was involved much more in expanding empire, in wars of trade, none of which threatened the social order to any great extent. In fact, imperial expansion, in combination with the Industrial Revolution, fed into the growth of wealth, markets, population and urbanization that characterized Queen Victoria's reign (Trevelyan 2000). The growth of cities thereby generated, and the wealth from 'trade', rather than inherited landowning, creating an aspirant middle class with very firm views on the social structure that have been well documented, not least by novelists such as Dickens and Trollope. In terms of how the powerful in that society then dealt with the poor, including disabled people, the former author is equally insightful, with the opening of *Oliver Twist* providing a graphic description of the iniquity of the workhouse that still has power to grip the modern reader.

With Darwin's work, as we have seen, many connections were made between the 'progress' of the industrialized nations, and the 'savagery' of the conquered countries, paralleled by the belief that the socially engendered class system was similarly a part of 'natural selection' (Churchill 1909). Quotations from Tredgold in Chapter 2 bring us back to intellectual disability, but do not really convey the link between an intellectual hierarchy and a social one which seems to me to be the peculiar feature of the English experience of eugenics, and to continue, in terms of attitudes to intellectual disability, to this day.

The twentieth century – eugenics and 'colonies'

With the extra twist of the class system, therefore, and politicians speaking quite openly about the 'lower orders', other events in intellectual disability services from the beginning of the twentieth century in England had all the elements that we have discussed in other chapters, following the same, earlier, educational optimism. The 1913 Mental Deficiency Act, strongly influenced by Tredgold and the eugenicists, laid down the classification of 'mental defect- ives' that was to last for over 50 years, including the controversial 'moral defective category' where people, often young women who got pregnant or young men who got drunk and involved in violence, could be certified as someone who 'from an early age display some permanent mental defect coupled with strong vicious or criminal propensities on which punishment has had little or no effect' (Mental Deficiency Act 1913 section 1).

The institutions that were either expanded from the 'asylums' of more optimistic times (Race 2002b), or built new, had all the features of such estab- lishments in the other countries, as well as being the model for a number of them in the colonies, and exporting people to run them. Ironically, however, English institutions were not called hospitals, but 'colonies', yet another unconscious reference, perhaps, to the superiority of the 'British race' over those put at a distance. Though they usually had a 'medical superintendent' and people called nurses, they were part of local government (now called Local Authorities – LA hereafter) provision, along with the still remaining workhouses. Some, indeed, were converted workhouses.

England also participated in the sterilization debates of the first part of the twentieth century, with the 'Eugenics Society' prominent among those calling for both sterilization and segregation of 'the unfit'. England never passed a law authorizing sterilization, but there is ample evidence (Fennell 1995) of its taking place, especially in the 'colonies' and especially for women.

Post-war changes – the NHS rules

'Colonies' in England were therefore much the same by the 1950s as contemporary institutions in the other countries. The administration of them,
however, had undergone an important change. The major welfare reforms of
the post-war Labour government included, in fact starred, the National
Health Service (NHS). Allocated to this national body, after some debate, were
the 'colonies' which became 'hospitals' overnight. The effect of this move,
with its concomitant inclusion of all grades of nursing, medical and ancillary
staff into the common pay scales, hierarchies, training and budgetary systems
of the NHS, cannot be over-emphasized, bringing with it the accumulated
wisdom and values of 40 years of segregation, including, as virtually the
only major textbook of its day, a further five editions of Tredgold's *Mental
Deficiency*. This needed continuously to be explained during my travels, since
in no other country was the power of the national Department of Health,
and the only *specialist* professional qualification being 'learning disability
nursing', at all comparable, or even comprehensible, given those countries'
post-normalization developments.

The immediate effects of the NHS takeover, again involving English class
issues, was the far higher status of the medical professions, giving greater
authority to the institutional regimes, and, because they were part of the popular 'free' health service, a perception of 'rightness' about them. This medical
credibility was incorporated into the next legal definition of intellectual disability, with the two categories of 'subnormal' and 'severely subnormal' using
the language of people being 'patients' (Mental Health Act 1959).

In education, too, the 1944 Education Act, setting up a supposed 'universal free' system of education, enshrined in law the existing practice
whereby a category of children were defined as 'incapable of receiving education at school'. These 'ineducable' children, defined as such by the IQ tests
that were also the basis of the selection of children at 'eleven plus' for the
'appropriate school', had no schools at all to attend. Controversy over the
'eleven plus', however, again endowing class status on the small proportion
(with a built-in gender bias in the system of allocation, Crook et al. 1999) of
those who got to grammar school, overshadowed the small voice of the
embryonic National Society for Mentally Handicapped Children in seeking to
get education for their offspring.

For parents of a child with intellectual disabilities, then, the 1950s and
1960s presented very similar options to pre-war, but with the status and
authority of the medical and educational professional establishment of the
welfare state. They could take what was usually the advice on the birth of a
child with an obvious condition, such as Down's syndrome, to 'leave them
here, and let the NHS look after them' or they could raise the child, without a
school to send them to, and with only the hospital as an alternative.

Normalization – an academic arrival

I have written elsewhere, Race (2002a) of the growth, within this dominant institutional culture, of a modest influence from academics, mostly psychologists, and we have also already noted the presence of one of them, Jack Tizard, in the network of academics and policy-makers involved with the origins of normalization. Their studies, the international network and publication of *Changing Patterns* (Kugel and Wolfensberger 1969) as well as Pauline Morris's (1969) highly critical sociological study of conditions in 35 subnormality hospitals, went along with a series of 'scandals' in particular hospitals to produce sufficient pressure for the Minister, Richard Crossman, to overcome substantial resistance from senior civil servants at the Department of Health and Social Security and add to his previous efforts to improve the conditions of hospitals by commissioning a policy document setting out plans for change (Crossman 1977). This document, entitled *Better Services for the Mentally Handicapped* (DHSS 1971), represented a significant acknowledgement of normalization ideas in government thinking, though without naming them. *Better Services* merely speaks, without reference, of 'current thinking' but goes on to propose a reduction by nearly half of the hospital population in the next ten years. It also proposes that LA services, then about to be unified under the heading of 'Social Services Departments', should provide residential and day care for adults not in hospital, including those discharged under its proposals. The details of their attempts to do this, with limited experience of intellectual disability, with entirely different budgetary systems to the NHS, with local political control in LAs but a national bureaucracy in the NHS, and with major debates in the 1970s about who should run and be employed in services for people with intellectual disabilities, is elaborated elsewhere (Race 2002b). As is the fact that in achieving a right to education of 'all children' in the Education (Handicapped Children) Act of 1970, the parents group, then called the National Society for Mentally Handicapped Children (showing what had become the more common label for intellectual disability) had realized one of its major campaigning goals. It had also, in its sponsorship of the 'Slough Experiment' (Baranjay 1971), demonstrated the 'radical' alternative to hospital provision in the form of the (usually 24-bedded) hostel. Notice, too, that there is no suggestion still of the parents' group setting up their own state-funded services, though some local societies had run 'Junior Training Centres' in the 1960s as an alternative for children denied school access.

The push of *Better Services* resulted in a considerable expansion of LA-provided hostels and so-called Adult Training Centres. These latter services had already existed prior to 1971, and were commented on favourably by Wolfensberger in his account of a European trip in the early 1960s, but now, rather than being in buildings converted from other uses, the capital availability saw a large number of purpose-built ATCs, with facilities for the sort of work that was going on at the time in factories and other uses of manual labour. Still segregated, and though with the avowed purpose of training people for 'real work', these centres, with many buildings still remaining to the present, were very much the equivalent of the sheltered workshops set up in the 1970s and 1980s in many countries of my journey.

In England, however, the debates, and the coming of normalization as an *idea*, with people bringing back word of projects such as ENCOR (Menolascino et al. 1968) were perhaps more influential on policy documents and government reports than in practice. In particular, what was seen at the time as a highly important government appointed 'Committee of Inquiry into Mental Handicap Nursing and Care' (known as the Jay Committee) used, in its final report (Jay Committee 1979), terms very close to the sort of language that had appeared in the *Normalization* (Wolfensberger 1972) book. The prime purpose, however, of the Jay Committee was to look at whether the 'care' of people with intellectual disabilities should be in the hands of nurses, or whether there was a need for a 'new caring profession'. Though, as we have seen in the other historical sections, experience from overseas indicated that the sort of community-based services indicated by normalization did not need nurses, the Jay Committee did not come firmly down on the removal of their dominance of the service system. Even the demonstrable ability of people with a general residential care background to run hostels, and to oversee the first ever group home in England (Race and Race 1979), did not swing the balance of power held by the medical and nursing professions. The incoming Conservative government under Margaret Thatcher, elected the same year, stalled on the Jay Report and, as Ryan notes, by 1981: 'The Jay report . . . a ground-breaking inquiry . . . had been quietly buried and with it the heated controversy and commitment to extra expenditure that the government was too anxious to avoid' (Ryan and Thomas 1987: 153). As for normalization, the next decade was to see its adoption and adaptation, sometimes to the point of unrecognizability, while at the same time much bigger forces were determining the fate of services.

Thatcherism – the English Jabberwock?

Many discussions have taken place on the effect of what came to be called 'Thatcherism'. Wherever the truth might lie, I found myself, as I noted in the Swedish chapter, contrasting the *similarity* of the welfare states of England and Sweden on my first visit in the 1970s with the major *differences* 30 years later, and concluding that much of what had changed in services for people with intellectual disabilities had much more to do with cultural changes in England stemming from the Thatcher years than it did with the influence of normalization in my country, important though that was.

As far as services and the welfare state were concerned, Thatcherism meant, on the one hand, a business-friendly government committed to reducing taxes, and on the social side a deep suspicion of welfare dependency and anything resembling a 'social approach'. Indeed, one of Mrs Thatcher's most famous quotes was that 'there is no such thing as society, only individuals and their families' (Thatcher 1987). In other words, to roll back the 'nanny state' and encourage people to stand on their own feet was what the country needed after 'years of socialism'. It is no coincidence, of course, that the Thatcher years overlap extensively with the Reagan presidencies, and that the neo-liberal economic forces begun in that era spread far beyond the shores of England. We have seen their effects in New Zealand and Australia, as well as the associated phenomenon of 'managerialism' to which we will return.

In the early 1980s, however, as the Thatcher government got into full cost-cutting stride, it faced an interesting paradox. On the one hand, expensive long-stay hospitals on valuable land were being criticized by the normalization movement and others, thus suggesting hospital closure as a profitable way to meet the demands of the field. At the same time, however, the political project to run down the power of Local Authorities (LAs) and bring more power into the centre (Cutler and Waine 1997), was at odds with a hospital closure programme that would increase the alternative, LA services. The LAs, for their part, saw the expense of their own long-stay institutions, the hostels, mounting, at a time of cuts in government financial support, yet the alternatives, especially in residential care in ordinary housing, appeared even more expensive. Thus while there began to appear some nationally known 'ordinary housing' projects, these were rare, and usually needed a voluntary agency, such as Barnardos in the north west of England, to be prepared to 'experiment' (Alaszewski 1986). Similarly, despite an influential report from the Kings Fund (1984) on daytime activity, which advocated more effort in finding real employment for people, such schemes were rare, especially as unemployment nationally was escalating.

Another political aim of the government, the rapid growth in providers of residential care from private and voluntary agencies as opposed to LA services, added to the mix (Hadley and Clough 1996). This aim was realized most powerfully in homes for elderly people, but expanded into intellectual disability services. As part of this, and getting involved in direct services on any scale for the first time, Mencap, the name now used by the parents' organization, set up a 'Homes Foundation' which started to open many 'ordinary houses', though initially these tended to be large houses of 10–12 beds with very strict admission criteria. Other examples of increasing non-public provision were private 'community' projects, often set up by groups of nurses from the closing hospitals, and many of which were in ordinary houses with less than four people (Emerson et al. 1999).

Arrangements to close hospitals, and the beginnings of a wider range of alternatives for a number of groups, thus developed. The coincidence of these primarily economic moves and the growth of the normalization movement, probably at its height in the mid to late 1980s (Race 1999), tended to result in the gradual introduction of a standard 'model' for residential care in terms of the 4–6-bedded 'ordinary house'. Though reducing their numbers, however, the continued financial power of the Department of Health as compared with shrinking LA budgets saw many institutions diminish slowly, despite attempts to transfer funds with patients and various forms of 'joint financing' between the two bureaucracies. Residential care in 'ordinary housing' also began to be provided within the NHS, with people thus still technically 'patients', despite normalization, or a certain version of it, becoming part of nurse training.

The bigger picture then again had its impact on services. Following the Griffiths Report (DoH 1988) and a resultant White Paper (DoH 1989), the final working out of the impact of growing social security spending and the growing private sector came in the NHS and Community Care Act of 1990 and subsequent guidance (Hudson, 1994). Though significant in terms of *organizational* change, the initial impact of the Act on the *sort* of services provided did not seem to alter the path that had been gaining pace in the 1980s, which was largely along the broad lines suggested by the normalization movement. The hospitals continued to close, the independent sector took up more and more provision of services, and the system began to move towards the situation described in the non-Scandinavian countries of this book, namely a diffuse range of provision, from extremely institutional to radical 'ordinary living'. No one sector, either publicly or privately provided services, had a monopoly of a particular point on that range The diffusion of services also had the effect of diluting the effect of normalization, compounded by academic criticism of the ideas, or at least how they had been interpreted and implemented in England (Brown and Smith 1992), and considerable confusion over the differences between it and Social Role Valorization. That story is elaborated elsewhere (Race 1999), but in terms of its effects on services, factional disputes in the 'movement', the growing power of the disability lobby, and the continuing fragmentation of service provision into the 1990s and the new millennium meant, in my view, that never again was a single set of ideas to have the same impact.

The 'New Labour' government, elected in 1997, while claiming it would reduce the impact of the welfare market, did not return the service system to its old monopoly of public provision. Nor, according to many commentators (Powell 2002) did it roll back the centralizing tendencies of the Thatcher government, and has had limited success in dealing with the mighty empire that is the Department of Health. Therefore the pattern, or more accurately the lack of a pattern, of services begun in the early 1990s became established as the norm. The review of services (DoH 1999), leading to *Valuing People*, however, and statements in that document itself, still reveal many services whose settings and practices would have been expected to have disappeared by the new millennium, had the rhetoric of the 1970s and onwards become reality. That pattern is overviewed in our normal summary table (Table 8.1).

Table 8.1   Schematic overview of 'services' that affect the lives of people with intellectual disabilities in England

'Service'	Service type(s)	Specialist or generic?	Formal organizational place
Pre-natal services	Mostly easy access to genetic counselling and abortion	Generic and specialist	NHS Primary Care Trust (PCT) provided Primary care services. Private and voluntary provision
Post-natal and early childhood services	Family advice, medical support, respite, early education	Generic clinical and LA services – some agency input specialist	PCTs, LA Children's and Education Departments, private and voluntary agencies
Non-educational services for children	Family advice, medical support, respite	Generic clinical and LA services – some agency input specialist	PCTs, LA Children's and Education Departments, private and voluntary agencies,
Education services – children and young adults	Primary and Secondary schools. Some 'all age' special schools, Colleges	Generic and specialist	Local Authorities Independent school trusts
Education services – adults	Colleges and universities	Mostly generic some specialist residential colleges	Independent organizations
Residential services – adults	Many in 'group living' – some in ordinary houses, some still in hostels or hospitals – few in individual arrangements – many still with parents/ other relatives	Largely specialist	Most in Agencies, LA Adult Social Care Services, NHS Trusts – Some public housing/ Housing Assn.

Daytime services – non-work	Small and large specialist day services usually accessing community and college resources Daytime in residence	Largely specialist	Most in Agencies or LA Adult Social Care Services – NHS Trusts only run a few specific day services
Daytime services – work	Some open employment (mostly p/t) – via Connexions or specialist supported employment service. Few through generic Jobcentres	Largely specialist Jobcentres generic	Connexions and most employment services LA-based Jobcentres part of national employment service
Leisure assistance	Mainly mainstream with agency support for use, usually as part of day services – few specialist leisure agencies	Largely specialist	As for non-work day services, leisure agencies usually independent
Advocacy services	Parent support agencies, individual Citizen Advocacy agencies, and campaigning organizations	Specialist	Independent organizations
Financial assistance	National Social Security benefits	Specialist within generic service	National Benefits agency – local offices
Parental 'support services'	Acting as all parents – 'In control' or Direct payments	Specialist, in that all children are different	Individual

Services for people with intellectual disabilities in England

Pre-natal services – clinical excellence?

Despite the debates on screening being held in all the countries of my trip, and despite policies in many countries promoting selective screening, I still received a surprised response from my hosts regarding the English legal position, where the provisions of the Abortion (Amendment) Act of 1990 allow abortion of a disabled foetus up to term. Despite the views of the disability movement, especially disabled women, regarding the image of disabled people that current practices represent (Morris 1991), the ever-increasing utilitarian position revealed by the growth of genetic research and the continued dominance of the medical profession seem to be what leads practice. The story of how Adam arrived in our life is one I have told many times, and a version has already appeared in print. Anonymized for the particular context, placing us in a different part of the country and changing names, and sometimes genders, of the protagonists, it nevertheless makes the point. Readers will guess who 'Joshua' is, who

> had been born . . . in a market town on the other side of the county. Had he been born some ten miles further north, in a city in the next county, there was a high probability that he would still have been with his natural parents. That city's Social Services Department had a reconciliation scheme that had a ninety per cent success rate in reuniting parents and disabled children who had initially been rejected. Had Joshua been conceived some twenty miles further south, in yet a third county and its major city, there was an equally high chance that he would not have been born at all. That city's university hospital was pioneering much wider use of amniocentesis than was then common, and had thus been doing a wider 'sweep' of mothers. Had Joshua's mother lived in that city there was a high chance she would have been selected for a test, and thus a high chance that he would have been aborted. As it was, the sleepy market town maternity hospital where he was born simply responded to the rejection of Joshua by his parents by placing him for adoption, some twenty-four hours after his birth.
>
> (Race 2002a: 230–1)

In the same chapter as that story is an account of a lecture discussing the ethical dilemmas faced by NHS-employed midwives, some ten years after Adam's birth, when they were largely responsible for having to give advice about the then new 'test' called chronio-vilius sampling. This test only suggests a *probability* of Down's syndrome, leading to a decision by the mother, if the probability is deemed 'high' whether to have a full amniocentesis and, if Down's syndrome is established, a termination. As we have seen, such tests are now commonplace, but ten or so years ago, when the Salford lecturer, in her job as a midwife, was asked to give 'advice and support', neither tests nor advice were uniform within the NHS, where the great bulk of services before and after the birth of a child in England are still found. She later sought the views of midwives on this issue, hence the lecture (ibid.: 229–30). The key issue concerned the sheer momentum of the process and the assumptions behind it, that having a child with Down's syndrome was automatically bad, and that as midwives, it was their duty to put that over to mothers. Those who adopted a broader counselling approach, sometimes with the result that mothers did not want to proceed with testing, often found themselves overruled by doctors the next time the mothers visited the hospital.

Since then, despite the much greater visibility of Down's syndrome in real communities and in the media, the position appears to be no better, in terms of the chances of Adam being born, were he to be conceived now. Much less dependent now on where his natural parents would be in the country, the advice of the National Institute for Clinical Excellence (NICE 2003) is that tests for establishing the probability of Down's syndrome should automatically be offered, with the assumption that an amniocentesis (or even a straight termin- ation) would follow if the test produced a 'bad result'. Set up in 1999 by the New Labour government, NICE is supposed to evaluate 'best practice' both in terms of efficacy and 'value for money'. Its views, though not mandatory, have usually been followed by NHS Primary Care trusts. It is therefore ironic that when, in 2003, it had just given its seal of approval for the automatic screening of all pregnant women for Down's syndrome, while at the same time reducing other antenatal checks, a curate from Chester, in the middle of England, was seeking a review of the decision not to prosecute doctors who aborted a child beyond the 24 weeks limit, when abortion is only permitted on the grounds of 'severe disability'. Her concern was that the 'severe disability' in question was a cleft palate. In the event she lost the case, on the grounds that doctors believed in good faith that there was a risk of severe disability.

So if Adam were conceived in England today, there would be a strong chance of his not being born.

Early childhood services – keeping the professionals employed

Comparing Adam's early childhood with the elements of the specific objec- tive in *Valuing People* brings to mind some interesting issues that were raised by the services we, and he, were offered in those pre-school days in the late 1980s:

> Objective 1: Disabled children and young people
> To ensure that disabled children gain maximum life chance bene- fits from educational opportunities, health care and social care, while living with their families or other appropriate settings in the com- munity where their assessed needs are adequately met and reviewed.
> (DoH 2001: 26)

Five years on from the White Paper, and comparing what appears to be offered now with what we received for Adam, my impression is that: (1) early child- hood services for all children are well provided, have numerous professional specialties, and have developed a degree of interdisciplinary working that was less common in the late 1980s, but (2) inclusion in mainstream services for children and families has become more varied, as the non-medical or therapeutic children's services have become dominated by the child protection agenda, and a backlash has begun in education. We will return to the latter, but would say that it is likely that, if Adam were born now, and leaving aside the adoption issue, we as parents would receive a good level of intervention from professionals in his early years. This we received in reality; paediatricians, health visitors, physiotherapists and our own GP were all involved, and had Adam been our natural son, then district nurses would also have been involved in his early months. Had Adam had more serious impairments, these professionals, all from the NHS and therefore all 'free', would have had a greater intensity of involvement, then as now. As it was, Adam had few of the specific health problems sometimes associated with Down's syndrome, and only his lack of conformity to the order of developmental stages by standing up before he could sit up occupied the concerns of these professionals. (The physiotherapists devised a fascinating device, like a corner shelf with a stick at the front of it that would jab Adam in the chest if he flopped forward. In the event, because he also showed much greater flexibility than the charts said he should have, he was able to wriggle out of it quite successfully and just sat up of his own accord in due course.)

On the less medical side, Adam also attended an integrated playgroup, was visited by a 'peripatetic education advisor' and went, as had his brothers, to a local state nursery school. We were fortunate that the latter provision existed in our area, as both state nursery schools (taking children from 3–5, before statutory school age) and rural schools in general were being intensively rationalized as the Thatcher government hit LA budgets (Pilcher and Wagg 1996). So Adam was fortunate in not only having such provision in our neighbouring village, but also that it was run by a person totally committed to take all children, and in a Local Authority Education area that had public commitment to inclusion.

Returning to other pre-school services it is clear from *Valuing People*'s references to the 'range of family support services' that such services existed in 2001, and were looking to be expanded. These were, of course, mostly services for *all* children, though they also included what have become known as Child Development Centres. Since 2001, the 'Surestart' policy (http://www.surestart.gov.uk/aboutsurestart/) has encouraged a move from separate centres for 'health', provided within the NHS system, and 'Children's Centres', LA-led facilities with a focus on social care, especially child protection, towards centres incorporating both aspects. Many 'children's teams' of health and social care professionals do now exist, despite the organizational differences, and within the intellectual disability part of the general process they seem to have a rather longer history of developing ways of working together, combining the continued use of early education schemes, such as Portage, (http://www.portage.org.uk/) which had already been around in Adam's time, and 'respite services' which continue to vary considerably in their nature, but with a lot more being home-based rather than institutional (Argent and Kerrane 1997), with access to developments, in the generic care system, of the increasing number (and increasing regulation and inspection) of childminders and nurseries.

As many professionals as were involved with Adam would therefore probably be around today. They would also be more likely, if they followed later education legislation (Education Act 2002), to assist us in finding inclusive nursery or pre-school provision, which we needed great fortune in our location and the particular moment in time to achieve for Adam. We would also, in theory, have more chance of getting him into mainstream education, which needed more than just fortune as we shall see next, after the 'Adam Back Home' box.

ADAM BACK HOME

Conceived in England – what next?

With developments in testing since Adam's birth in 1985, and the great majority of pregnant women using NHS maternity services, the NICE guidelines would almost certainly mean we would be offered one or other of the tests that give a probability of Down's syndrome, with an assumption of amniocentesis and termination if we had a 'bad' result. Therefore, Adam would have less chance of being born in England than was the case in 1985. Though we, as parents, would be more aware of Down's syndrome, the views expressed in that greater awareness, especially in the media, would not tend to make us likely to refuse the offer of tests. If Adam were born, however, initiatives for children in general, together with the sort of basic health care and early childhood work for disabled children that was around when Adam was actually born, would probably mean a greater chance of his being involved in inclusive childcare settings, such as Children's Centres. Other services, which may be based at the Children's Centres or exist in their own right, could be early education schemes, such as Portage, and we would expect to find childminders or nurseries that would be inclusive. We might also be able to enrol Adam at a nursery school (the one he actually went to still survives, unlike many rural schools following the Thatcher years) and begin the 'statementing process' by which his educational future would be decided. This process would begin, in any case, before mandatory school age for someone like Adam, with an obvious intellectual disability, and even were his disability less obvious, many of the generic services mentioned above would have raised issues with us, especially if we were middle-class articulate parents.

Education, education, education – inclusion at the crossroads?

The famous mantra of Tony Blair prior to the 1997 election may now be coming back to haunt him for other reasons than inclusion, though the subject did appear to be the only time intellectual disability was raised as he went for a third term in 2005. This occurred when the mother of a child with autism cornered the Prime Minister in a TV studio discussion and refused to let him move until he had answered her question regarding what she perceived as the lack of support her son was getting because of the 'inclusion policy' of the government. Certainly, point (4) of *Valuing People* Objective 1 (2001: 122) reveals the degree to which 'education in inclusive settings in their own communities' is perceived to be 'best practice', and, of course, 'Inclusion', is one of the four 'key principles' of the White Paper as a whole. Blair's encounter with the parent in 2005, however, together with the construction of new 'special schools' in recent years, suggest that there may be the beginnings of a backlash against inclusive education. The government's 2005 Education Bill, published while I was away, gives implicit confirmation of this trend, in terms of proposals for the expansion of 'specialist academies' of different kinds, in such things as sport, the arts, etc., but also what would be in effect 'specialist special schools'.

So how different is it from the process of 'statementing', introduced in the 1981 Education Act, and applied to Adam as he was coming up to school age in the late 1980s. As we have seen, he was by then attending his local state nursery school, and at that point had no specific extra assistance at school, though he was visited and had sessions with a person known as a 'peripatetic special education advisor', employed by the LA Special Needs Section.

Ten years earlier, a key government report in the eventful year of 1979, the Warnock Report, reflected developments in many countries by proposing 'integrated education'. Its recommendations were largely adopted in the 1981 Education Act, including the process by which children identified as potentially having 'special educational needs' were to have a 'statement' of these needs put together by the LA, in consultation with parents and all relevant professionals. The statement pronounced on what *sort* of schooling would best meet those needs, then suggested a specific school where this might occur. It is important to remember here that well over 90 per cent of schools at this time were funded and administered by LAs, taking up a large proportion of their overall budgets. Suggestions of schools in a statement, then, very much depended on the LA's attitude to inclusion, its provision of 'special schools', and its overall financial health. As we have mentioned, by the time Adam came up to 4, budgets of LAs had been severely cut, and, like the de-institutionalization process being a coincidence of radical views and political expediency for the government, so the closure of special schools and the reduction of 'Special Needs sections' by LAs coincided with growing academic and other support for inclusion. Educational psychologists, employed by LAs, were the co-ordinators of the statementing process, and when all the various professionals, including the Head of the nursery school and the peripatetic advisor, declared that Adam's needs could be met in a mainstream school, it was difficult for the educational psychologist, who had met Adam a couple of times, to disagree. What he could do, however, was to suggest that, rather than attend the small village school, which acted as an 'infants school' (ages 5–7) and fed into a larger primary school (ages 5–11) in the nearby town, Adam should be part of a 'Special Needs Unit' in a primary school some 10 miles away. Thus instead of going to the school where his brothers had, and did, attend, with other children of the village, Adam would be 'taxied' to the other school. Since the taxi had to pass through the playground of the other school, it would have to arrive earlier, and leave later, than the buses bringing the other children, none of whom would have come from our village in any case. Our suspicions of ulterior motives, and source of many later stories, were raised by visiting the 'unit'. Space does not permit the many attributes that enabled this visit to be a model, in future SRV presentations, for demonstrating the devaluation process, but key to motives was the fact that the 'unit' was not full, and the only way the LA was likely to save on costs and reduce special school numbers was to demonstrate its 'financial viability'.

Memories of the subsequent meeting are hazy, but at one point, when Debbie's anger against the recommendation became obvious, the educational psychologist suggested that she had not come to terms with having a disabled child. This not only revealed a lack of depth in his enquiries, but turned the meeting somewhat our way when we revealed Adam was adopted. Eventually, therefore, we succeeded in getting the recommendation changed, to read that Adam should attend the village school, and have an 'Educational Care Officer' (ECO) employed on a part-time basis to support him.

Before we compare Adam's actual time at school with what might be provided now, a brief comment on the current statementing process is in order. Though amended in detail by subsequent Education Acts, the basic pro-cess seems the same. The key difference appears to be that the role of the LA has become more one of co-ordinating the process, rather than having as much effect as previously on the choice of school. In the later years of the Conservative government, the role of governors of schools (lay volunteers elected by parents), and their degree of autonomy over budgets and admis-sions policy changed considerably. At the same time the introduction of a National Curriculum and national testing of children at various ages in 1988 led to 'league tables' of schools. Combined with broader social change, this has meant education has evolved into the sort of 'quasi market' that emerged in other parts of the welfare state (Bartlett et al. 1998). Accepting a child with Down's syndrome would, of course, have some effect on the league tables, continued by the incoming New Labour government, who added other parameters for classifying schools as part of their 'drive to raise standards' (Powell 2002) and 'increasing choice'. The new processes still have the presumption of inclusion as the norm, but their playing out in practice has now become much more variable (Rustemier and Vaughan 2005).

So were Adam coming up to 5 today, he would still be statemented, and in somewhere as small and rural as our village and surrounding area, options would depend largely on the attitude of the various schools. He would still be likely to be offered a place at a mainstream primary school, though attempts to close the local special school have not come to fruition, and we as parents would still have to be firm, but when it came to secondary school the options would be much more dependent on where we lived, and which primary school Adam had attended.

As it was, once Adam had got into the village school, his performance, and the hard work of his teachers, led to far fewer difficulties moving on to the town primary school when he reached 7. In turn, the experiences of each year's class teacher, with help from excellent ECOs and the headteacher, who moved from a deep sceptic to the fiercest advocate of inclusion, led to a very positive case being made for him to go to the main secondary school in the town, attended already by two of his brothers. Adam's development as a pupil, of course, also played a part, and space does not permit the many stories contained in the years described by those brief sentences. A number of them are, naturally, about difficult times as well as moments of tear-jerking joy, but they add up to the bald fact that Adam took part in the mainstream curriculum, with support for a good part of his day from the ECO.

He moved at 11 to the secondary school, achieved with much less difficulty than the village school admission, with only the educational psychologist – not the same one – suggesting the possibility of a special school place, and her part in the process was much less powerful at this stage. Early focus on which subjects in the national examinations Adam might succeed in meant he had something of a modified curriculum at secondary level, but not one solely for him, in that he shared some extra reading and maths lessons with a smaller 'remedial' group. The main other issue that came up was bullying, which was dealt with very well by the school, and in an ironic way it was fortunate that the school had a wider bullying problem at the time, since Adam's issues could be dealt with as part of an overall strategy, rather than singling him out.

In Emerson et al.'s 2003/4 survey of just under 3,000 adults (defined as over 16), (Emerson et al. 2005), 72 per cent had been to a special school, 10 per cent to a special unit in a mainstream school and 18 per cent to ordinary classes in mainstream school. Discounting the data from older adults, some of whom had not been to school at all, the figures over the 33 years since the 1970 Education Act (i.e. data for under-45s) did not show a dramatic or consistent rise in inclusion. Being younger and having lower support needs were the only variables associated with people having gone to a mainstream school, and these data support the view that were Adam now of school age, he would still have the odds against him being as fully included as he was.

In the event he succeeded in passing six of the public examinations (known as GCSEs) at 16, achieving more passes than some of his non-disabled contemporaries (and six more than his footballing hero, David Beckham) and so left school.

Had he been in a special school, ironically, he would have been assumed to continue until 19. Not because he might take the next 'Advanced level' examinations, the usual reason for pupils staying beyond 16 at mainstream schools; in fact, had he been at special school, the chance of his even taking GCSEs would have been slim; nor in order to get significantly involved in vocational training. He would have stayed on at special school simply because that is how such schools developed, with many still taking 'children' right through from 5 to 19, though there are a few 'sixth form colleges' that are separate from the pre-16 group. The assumption of the English educational system, very much influenced by the relative value given to vocational and academic subjects, is that most school leavers from mainstream schools will either go straight into work (in low wage-type employment) or go to what are known as 'Further Education (FE) colleges' where they can take more vocational courses in things like plumbing, carpentry or hairdressing. Again it is hard to describe to outsiders the class associations that go along with these options.

So Adam went to FE college, but not to a specifically vocational subject. Instead, joining the 19 and 20-year-olds from the special school leavers (and older students repeating the course for the third or fourth time), he became part of the 'Learning for Living' course, a segregated programme at the far end of the college (next to the large dustbins 'for ease of access of the dustcarts') whose students shared some of the same general facilities as the trainee carpenters, hairdressers and caterers but little in the way of teaching.

Now, five years after Adam's college entry, the position would be much the same, despite *Valuing People*'s objectives regarding 'transition'. The process of 'transition review' is a legally mandated procedure, supposed to be person-centred and take place in a co-ordinated way between the various 'stakeholders', beginning at school when pupils are 14, and then updated annually until they leave. Its intention is to smooth the path from the world of children's services, especially the all-embracing nature of the school system, to the adult world, for which read adult services. The overwhelming focus on *academic* achievement in schools, however, means that those at the lower end of the intellectual hierarchy get rather less attention, as for most of them there is the well-founded assumption that they will leave at 16 and get a job. For those right at the bottom, i.e. people with intellectual disabilities, they will either be in special schools, where a whole different set of assumptions reign, with very little dependence on academic achievement to move to the next stage in the service path, or oddities, like Adam, who have made it to mainstream schools but are unlikely to be able to walk into a job at 16. In recent years, probably the last ten or so, colleges and 'Learning for Living' type courses have taken most special school leavers, and 'transition' reviews predominantly lead to that pathway. Emerson et al.'s survey again is illustrative. Of the 928 people they interviewed who were under 25, 52 per cent were attending school or college, with 36 per cent of people of all ages currently doing some kind of course or training, mostly at colleges.

So the transition review process tends to produce a predictable path for people with intellectual disabilities, much as it was in when Adam left school.

ADAM BACK HOME

Going to school in England

Though, in most places, we would have begun the 'statementing process' for Adam before mandatory school age, since his intellectual disability would have been picked up well before he was a 'rising five', this would not necessarily be the case for others with less obvious disabilities. Whether the process would then have started before school age varies with both the location and the class of us as parents, and how 'pushy' we were. Class and location, especially in urban areas of England, tend to be highly correlated, with schools in areas of large public housing (known as 'council estates') tending to be most likely to take children who would subsequently go through the statementing process, whereas the more middle-class or mixed areas would have a number of parents who would have been involved with services if their child had even mild signs of intellectual disability. Eventually, assuming the child has an intellectual disability, the statement and educational plan will be formulated. If we pushed for mainstream schooling for Adam, our chances of success would again vary with our location, the degree to which the LA was committed to inclusion (or had inherited a situation of no special schools) and the attitude of the particular school Head and/or governors. The odds are still against inclusion, even more so against full inclusion, and a great deal depends as well on how persistently we present the case, increasingly too on whether we go to law. If we take what we are given, then again local circumstances will affect Adam's inclusion, but it would be more likely to occur at primary school level than secondary. If he went to a special school, however, that would probably be where he would stay from 5-19. If Adam were at mainstream, some schools would try (as the real one did) to get him through the public GCSEs at 16, others would try to line him up with employment, some would do both, but the most likely outcome from school would be his going to college, where he would join the school leavers from the special schools. This would be difficult to avoid, even if we wanted him to get into employment on leaving school, ironically more so if he had been to mainstream and thus left at 16, and even if the transition review process had been fully carried out. Developments in person-centred approaches at the school level, using this review process, might be our only variation from the inexorable route to college, especially if our LA was involved in the development of individualized funding. As we shall see, however, this would not apply to Adam at present, given his competence and our lack of 'crisis' in supporting him.

Daytime services – work or occupation?

The prevalence of college placements in England, noted above, has continued since Adam's school leaving five years ago, despite government objectives, expressed in *Valuing People*, for both a 'modernization' of day services and extra efforts to get people into employment. The part played by colleges in this is assumed to be concerning employment, their role for the majority of the non-disabled students, and this was our hope, if not expectation, for Adam. In the event, though his college experience had a lot of benefits for his social life, especially his first close relationship, in terms of preparing him for employment, or even in fact maintaining his level of basic academic skills, we saw very little progress.

Objective 7 of *Valuing People* includes the statement 'To enable people with learning disabilities to lead full and purposeful lives within their community and to develop a range of friendships, activities and relationships' (DOH 2001: 76). Acknowledging their chaotic state, *Valuing People* requires LAs to draw up plans to 'modernize' day services by 2006. A small amount of seed money was on offer, with day services being a priority for the Learning Disability Development Fund, and the new Learning Disability Partnership Boards being required to draw up modernization programmes by 2002, including addressing the future role of existing large day centres. Other factors, however, have militated against such plans being implemented. First is the FACS criteria (DoH 2003), whose levels, as then codified by individual LAs, meant that legally *required* services came first, and then usually only for the top two criteria of 'critical' and 'substantial', leaving those whose needs were considered 'moderate' or 'low'. Since day services are not clearly legally mandated, and many people attending them are not in the top two categories, many LAs simply held on to their buildings and tried to do whatever they could in terms of 'community involvement' with these as a base, though some used bases in more generic community centres, or widened the client group of the intellectual disability centres (Valuing People Support Team 2005).

In Adam's case, there was no contact with the main day service system until he had been at college for a couple of years, for the simple reason that he was not legally an adult until then. What we had done, once it became clear that no real work possibilities looked like emerging from the college, was to discover that an experimental 'supported employment' service was being set up in our part of the county, funded in part by European Union initiatives on employment of disabled people. So, as Adam passed 18, he was beginning to be supported at work, first in the village shop and then in a small shop in the nearby town, in the two days that he was not at college. We will return to this part later, when we look at employment services, but continuing Adam's experiences of day services other than employment, we jump three years ahead. In 2005, he began attending, one day per week, the day service in another town about 6 miles away from our village. This service, like a number that had closed or moved from large centres, was based at a community centre in the town, but mainly focused on community activities outside the building. They did, however, have a specialist art teacher, who ran one half-day session aiming at producing quality art work, and this was the key reason for Adam attending. It would be fair to say that the service has been a positive experience for Adam, especially with the art programme, though we are perhaps a little more critical of the 'community activities' offered in the rest of his day, which basically consists of bussing a group of four or five about 15 miles to a larger town to go bowling. As for how typical Adam's current experience is, judging from both personal observation and the literature, he has been lucky to even get one day per week (and even luckier, some six months ago, to get two, which he currently has). Many authorities have stuck more rigidly to the FACS criteria than Derbyshire, an observation borne out by Emerson et al. (2005).

Remembering the figures for college attendance from their survey (36 per cent of the whole survey and 52 per cent of the under-25s), the figure of 39 per cent of their interviewees who said they went to a day centre seems much lower than would have been the case ten or more years ago. In addition, the fact that, of the people who did go to a day centre, only 42 per cent went for five days a week, with similar numbers of the remainder going one, two, three or four days a week, confirms the sort of variation in quantity and quality of provision noted above. It might also be a sign that more people are getting into employment, but both Adam's experiences and other data suggest that, though there has been some growth, it has been slow and very patchy.

Employment services and person-centred approaches – individual solutions, but for how many?

The practice of the supported employment scheme, though new to our area, will be familiar to many people in the countries I visited, with a worker being attached to Adam, working alongside him initially so that the employer was assured of the tasks being carried out, and then gradually withdrawing. Given its experimental nature, and the fact that there were only two people involved at the outset, it took some months before the process described above began, but this expanded to the point where Adam was working three days a week as a cleaner in an outdoor centre run by the LA. 'Workstep', a scheme to assist people who have difficulty accessing employment (http://www.jobcentreplus. gov.uk/JCP/Customers/Helpfordisabledpeople/Workstep/index.html), then contributed to the support worker and transport for Adam, as the centre was a few miles outside of the nearest town. Eventually, the centre was able to offer Adam the job on a paid basis, and he has been in the employ of the LA for nearly three years as this is written.

Given that *Valuing People* made employment a specific objective, with other day services consolidated under the objective quoted above, Adam could therefore be thought of as a successful example of government policy. Certainly other action in the broader context of the 'welfare to work' agenda of the government, especially tax credits, but also the specific 'Action point' (2001: 85) from *Valuing People* that 'Disabled people starting work will not lose Disability Living Allowance unfairly', led to a situation where Adam could be employed for 20 hours a week, not lose benefit, and claim tax credit. This almost put him in a position where he was receiving an income equivalent to a full-time worker. Again, however, many factors had to coincide to achieve the above state of affairs; our good fortune in the new programme starting up; Adam still being confident in his abilities from his school experience; the extra motivation gained by meeting a girlfriend at college and hoping to move from home and be with her; our desire to get Adam into work; and our knowledge of the human service system. For Adam's contemporaries in our area, who had mostly gone to special school and college, the notion of work was not really on the agenda, and though some attempts were made at work placements within the college course, lack of staff and a specific budget for this activity meant that prospects of success were limited. This concurs with Emerson et al.'s findings, that for most people, adult day services, or the lack of them, are what they are presented with, rather than employment. In that survey, 29 per cent of interviewees were not involved with *any* of the three daytime activities of work, education/training, or day centre, while 17 per cent had a paid job and 6 per cent had an unpaid job. Many who did have paid jobs worked part-time, with 28 per cent of men and 47 per cent of women working less than 16 hours a week (Emerson et al. 2005: 55–8). Adam's experience of the *sort* of work he was offered, i.e. shop work or cleaning, is also reflected in Emerson et al.'s survey (ibid.: 48) with that type of work figuring in the five most frequent categories. Adam's best 'work experience' at school was in a solicitor's office, but only 2 per cent of those in jobs were involved in office work.

It is clear, therefore, and supported by other sources, that though Objective 8 of *Valuing People* couldn't be clearer when it wishes. 'To enable more people with learning disabilities to participate in all forms of employment, wherever possible in paid work, and to make a valued contribution to the world of work' (DoH 2001: 26), the progress five years later is limited (Valuing People Support Team 2005). When Emerson et al.'s (2005) survey is further consulted, we find 62 per cent of those not in work claiming this is because they 'Cannot work or nobody would employ them because they have a disability' and yet 65 per cent said they would like a job. The difficulty we have found in other countries regarding real work seems to be equally true for England.

Of note here, and also as a link to the world of residential services, the role of 'person-centred approaches' needs to be discussed, and another aspect of Adam's experience used to put it into focus. The phrases 'person-centred approaches', and 'person-centred planning' often occur in *Valuing People*, such as in the day service discussion where 'The introduction of person-centred planning for people using day centres will be a key element for achieving . . . modernisation. People using them should be an early priority for person-centred planning' (DoH 2001: 78). Such was the commitment to these approaches that an extensive guide, with a range of tools, methodologies and references was issued just under a year later (Valuing People website). The difficulty, however, of using such individualized methods in systems geared to bulk contracts and overall planning, with co-operation between different service funding and delivery systems at the abstract and number-led level of strategic management, soon became apparent (Race, D.M. 2006).

Our experience with Adam is not typical, but does illustrate some issues, especially about the difficulty of adult services to share and co-ordinate action, and the ubiquity of assessment, rather than action, in the lives of those involved. At our instigation, in 2003, a group of people involved with Adam came together for a PATH (Pearpoint et al. 1993) meeting. Though it was facilitated by someone internationally known for pioneering such approaches, the participants from the service side of things had not only never heard of our facilitator, but had no experience of this form (or any form, as far as we could see) of person-centred planning. Because we had arranged it ourselves, the PATH meeting had no authority behind it, though it was extremely useful for focusing Adam's mind on what he wanted to do, and its immediate 'service' effects were confined to Adam being offered a few days of 'respite care' as it was officially called, as a 'practice' for him moving out to live independently. Achieving even this limited amount of service involved more 'assessments'. Prior to the PATH, Adam had already been assessed, separately, for college, for the supported employment scheme, and for a voluntary 'leisure service' (though the latter got no further than the assessment). Once Adam turned 18, he was then entitled under the 1990 NHS and Community Care Act to an official assessment of his needs by the LA. Though far more comprehensive and personal (and one of the processes mentioned in the DOH guidance), the PATH meeting could not be a substitute. Nor could the LA assessment suffice for all the 'respite care' houses subsequently attended by Adam, since two were provided by the local NHS trust. For these, we had to spend a morning visiting the psychiatric consultant and the nurse in charge of the first 'respite' house. This was despite the NHS trust service being provided in very similar building, with very little observable difference in staffing or activities, to the 'respite house' that resulted from the LA assessment, and the only reason Adam wanted to go there was because his girlfriend also went there, though they never actually got to attend together.

The social worker at the time of the PATH moved on soon afterwards, and was not replaced for a while, a not unusual event in LA Social Services Departments, and it was only an attempt, two years later, by her successor to check on her own caseload before she, too, left for another job that put us back in touch with Social Services. Though that worker did leave, she set in train a meeting with *her* successor, at which point the need for something else for Adam than college was uppermost in our, and his, minds. After undertaking yet another assessment meeting (no record of the PATH or the original LA assessment seemingly having been kept), the daytime place for Adam noted above was finally agreed – one day per week, specifically for the art session.

So the result of our 'person-centred plan', the PATH meeting, was largely one of Adam clarifying in his mind that he needed to work, which was already in train, that he needed to have time 'trying out' being away from home, which eventually came via nights and weekends in three different 6-bedded respite care homes, and that his dream of moving out with his girlfriend to set up home together could actually happen. The fact that he did eventually move out, though not with his girlfriend, had a lot to do with the thoughts that were focused at that meeting, and very little to do with the many assessments of his needs that still appear to be necessary before any service can be offered. Ironically, however, though not resulting from any service system processes, still less with any *official* 'person-centred plan', Adam's move could be said to have met the *Valuing People* objective for housing, as we shall see below.

Residential services – an ordinary house is not necessarily a home

In a comparison of the only two White Papers specifically to do with intellectual disability, namely *Valuing People* and the 1971 *Better Services* document (Race 2007), one of the key differences highlighted is the specific number and type of services proposed by the older document, as opposed to the mostly broad and unspecific targets in *Valuing People*. This is illustrated in miniature by Objective 6, on housing, and its three sub-objectives, abbreviated below

> Government objective: To enable people with learning disabilities and their families to have greater choice and control over where and how they live.
>
> • Increasing the range and choice of housing open to people with learning disabilities in order to enable them to live as independently as possible.
> • Ensuring people with learning disabilities and their families obtain advice and information about housing from the appropriate authorities.
> • Enabling all people currently in NHS long-stay hospitals to move into more appropriate accommodation and reviewing the quality of outcomes for people living in NHS residential campuses.
>
> (DoH 2001: 126)

The 'target' attached to the third sub-objective, of closing all the remaining long-stay hospital provision by 2004, is one of the few prescriptive statements in *Valuing People*, and, sadly, has still to be met (Valuing People Support Team 2005). The 'options for housing' given in *Valuing People* also suggest that the legacy of institutions is still alive and well, with 'Village and intentional communities', being named alongside 'Supported living', and 'Small scale ordinary housing' (DoH 2001: 73). The DoH nail their colours firmly to the fence in terms of not stating preferences, nor even claiming that these three are the only 'good practice' options. Despite the supposed 'dominance' of the normalization/SRV movement in England, and the 'inclusion' principle of *Valuing People*, segregated and congregated settings are still sanctioned. This also seems to represent current reality, with Emerson et al.'s survey, research done for the *Inclusion Europe* report (Freyhoff et al. 2004) and, on a personal scale, Adam's experience, confirming the continuing existence of the range of residential services that we have seen in most other countries of this book. Despite some notable individual achievements in 'supported living' in England, e.g. Harker and King (1999), the overwhelming impression remains that the congregate form of living, whether in 'ordinary houses' or larger institutions, is still the norm. In physical terms, things are certainly a lot further on, though far from the goal of normalization/

SRV and its successors for housing that does not adversely image the residents. Most people now live in domestic dwellings, but in terms of social integration the picture is far less rosy, as Davies and Spencer sum up succinctly:

> We think too few people (less than one in seven) live on their own or with a partner. Too many young people still live with their parents and too many older people live in supported accommodation. Living independently makes many choices possible but, just like everyone else, people with learning difficulties worry about safety in the area they live in. We don't think this should stop people living independently. They should have the choice of being independent and safe.
>
> (Davies and Spencer 2005: 27)

Adam's experience of 'respite care' being the only means services could offer him to 'practise' living away from home shows how difficult it appears to be for services to get out of the group home mindset. The fact that even this congregate form of living became unavailable to Adam, on the LA side, because financial pressures and the FACS criteria meant that the houses were only used for 'critical' people and not those who had 'chosen' to leave home, also shows why the numbers of people living at home remains high. Emerson et al. found 69 per cent of their survey living in 'private households' which they define as living alone, with a partner or with parents or other relatives. Of this group, 89 per cent were living with parents or other relatives, the great majority with the former, while 4 per cent lived with a partner (Adam's dream) and 6 per cent on their own. Of the people living with their parents, remembering that all were over 16, the age at which young people are legally allowed to leave home, 20 per cent had parents who were 65 or older, and 9 per cent had parents who were 75 or older.

The remaining 31 per cent of Emerson et al.'s interviewees therefore lived in some form of staffed accommodation, with 75 per cent of them living in houses for four or more people, 22 per cent in houses for more than ten people, and just 14 per cent in two or one person households. Some 67 per cent of this group 'said they had no choice (or were reported to have no choice) over who they lived with' and 54 per cent 'said they had no choice (or were reported to have no choice)' over where they lived (Emerson et al. 2005: 46). So even if the housing objective in *Valuing People* is excused from being specific about what might be good places for people to live, on the grounds of 'choice', that defence also falls down for a great many people. Using a definition of 'not enough choice' in housing being people who had *no choice* over *either* who they lived with *or* where they lived, Emerson's group found nearly two-thirds (64 per cent) of those in staffed accommodation did not have enough choice. So the picture is still one where the aspirations of both the normalization/SRV movement for 'full social integration' and of the social model adherents for 'rights' to choose where and with whom people live have met with limited success.

Adam's story comes fully up to date in the next section, alongside discussion of the success, again relative, of individualized initiatives. Both are about 'real life, not a service', one of the catchphrases of the latest of such initiatives.

Parents, advocates and supporters – who is 'In control'?

The culture of the welfare state, developed since the early twentieth century and in full swing after the Second World War, still has a deep impact on many people in England. On the other hand, the dismantling of significant parts of that welfare state and the promotion of independent agencies as the providers of services resulting from the Thatcher government seem to have gone along with the sharpening of the competitive elbows of English society which that same government released. This means, in my view, that parents still expect the state, be it local or national, to provide services for people with intellectual disabilities, but are also caught up with the increasing consumerist orientation of much of what were previously thought to be expectations of citizenship. Our experiences with Adam confirm this confusion. Where we want services to deal with *him*, and try to maximize *his* choices, we find that we still get 'letters home' asking our permission for various things. On the other hand, decisions that we would expect to have at least an input to, especially if they relate to resources, get taken without consultation because they are 'Adam's choice'. As it has turned out, the determination to live out at least some version of the dream brought out by the PATH process, and the confidence gained from dealing with people (including, but not only, his parents) who have consistently high expectations of him have enabled Adam to take advantage of circumstances in his real world, as opposed to his service-defined world, and make some choices that will have a significant effect on his life. Quite simply, a combination of our financial circumstances, his brother returning from university with a desire to live in our village if at all possible, and a two-bedroom house becoming available in the village has led to Adam and his brother moving into a place of their own. The first element of the combination is, perhaps, the most significant practically, in that we were able to raise money to lend to our sons, enabling them to own the property. Though there are a number of schemes (see http://www.housingoptions.org.uk/gi_publications.html, for example) by which people with intellectual disabilities have been enabled to buy their own homes, their low level of paid employment and the general boom in house prices that continues to go unabated in England mean that the number of people in such circumstances is small. No mention is made of whether any of Emerson et al.'s (2005) interviewees owned or part-owned their accommodation, though it would not be unreasonable to assume that the great majority of those living with parents or in residential care homes do not.

Adam is therefore in a fortunate position, both in terms of the availability of accommodation in the village where he has become a member of the community in his own right, but also in earning sufficient income to repay his half share of the house. The move came as something of a surprise to Adam's social worker, when we mentioned it as an aside to supporting Adam's request for an extra day at the day service, but she visited soon after and appeared satisfied that he was managing well enough. Over the years since the PATH meeting and the early experiences of 'respite' as practice for Adam moving out, we had used residential services relatively little, mainly when we were on holiday and none of his brothers were home. We had also begun to leave Adam on his own overnight if we were away somewhere, subsequently extending this to weekends. Adam had dealt with this very well, again a tribute to his confidence and abilities, so the move out was a logical step.

There is one current development in England (in fact, UK-wide) that might enable others to achieve a similar result. This is an initiative called *In Control*, begun in 2003 by a small group in the North-west of England, but quickly taken up by the *Valuing People* Support Team (VPST) nationally, and then financially supported as a series of pilot schemes by VPST and Mencap. It represents perhaps the most influential result of actions subsequent to *Valuing People*, both in terms of its effect on government policy and on the development of individualized funding, though as yet the full impact on a significant number of people has to be realized.

Citizen Advocacy, perhaps the only remotely comparable service focused on individuals, has had a somewhat chequered history in England, starting with the same energy as normalization, but getting tangled up with the tensions of the self-advocacy and self-determination debates we have noted in other countries (Race 2003). *In Control* which claims to pull together what it describes as the 'inclusion movement' and the 'independent living movement' may have a greater chance of success. Attempts at individualized funding, known as 'Direct Payments', were introduced some years ago for a range of social care services, especially those involving physically disabled people, partly as a result of the 'independent living' movement that social model adherents had been actively, and successfully promoting. The Community Care (Direct Payments) Act of 1996 could be set alongside the 1995 Disability Discrimination Act as achievements of this movement, though in both cases there have been issues of their significance for people with intellectual disabilities (Chappell 1998). Where Direct Payments have been awarded to people, they receive the cash equivalent of services they would otherwise be entitled to receive from LAs, or agencies funded by LAs, measured in terms of the actual cost of those services. Recipients (or their representatives) then managed those funds to pay for their support. In Emerson et al.'s survey, however, only 38 per cent of those interviewed had even heard about Direct Payments (2005: 7). The key shift in *In Control* is that an assessment of finance takes place first, before the *service form* by which the money is spent is determined. The *In Control* website (http://www.in-control.org.uk/home.php) gives more detail on how this exercise, known as the Resource Assessment System (RAS) is carried out but basically the disabled person fills out a questionnaire which assesses the impact of someone's disability on their life. Their answers generate a points total which is multiplied by a local 'price point'. The amount of a price point is worked out by each local authority individually based on its current pattern of expenditure.

Once the 'price points' for a person are realized in terms of a sum of money, a person-centred planning process takes place, to work out what support the person needs to live a 'real life'. This might include buying support from existing services, but also can involve the hiring of support workers, paying for generic services, or even hiring people to undertake tasks for parents or other family members so that they can have the time to support the person in particular aspects of their lives. *In Control* was originally piloted in six LAs on a voluntary basis, and reviewed in 2006 (Sanderson et al. 2006) by which time a larger network of organizations were responsible for the project, which has spread to some 85 LAs. It has also had a considerable effect on wider government policies. The review confirms the accounts of others (Morris 2005; Race 2005) of its influence, on three recent policy documents. The earliest of these, *Improving the Life Chances of Disabled People* (Cabinet Office 2005) citing *In Control* significantly, introduced to the wider policy field the notion of individual budgets, which was applied yet more widely in proposals for change in all forms of adult social care in the Green Paper, *Independence, Well-being and Choice* (DOH 2005), and confirmed in a third policy paper, *Opportunity Age* (DWP 2005). A government pilot Individual Budget Programme was initiated for two years from January 2006 in 13 LAs, each developing systems to deliver individual budgets over a two-year period. One of these, Oldham, is using *In Control* as its system for *all* adult social care.

The *In Control* review's overall conclusions suggest that disabled people and their supporters, when offered the chance, quickly demonstrate their capacity to take control and to make the most effective use of the community's funding of social care. This leads me to reflect that, as has been the case throughout this book, the closer 'services' can get to real life, the more they are in accord with what I draw from my years of involvement with the normalization/SRV network, and the nearer to the lessons I have learnt from having Adam as my son. That reflection should not be read as an opinion that England has found the Holy Grail of services via *In Control*. The government goal of a total take-up of individualized budget systems by 2012 will be a process fraught with difficulty, especially as the continuing troublesome marriage of NHS and LA systems and finances (only a small amount of NHS finance can currently be used for *In Control*) has been significantly affected by current government demands on PCTs to achieve balanced budgets (Carvel 2006).

Local politicians and their bureaucratic advisors will need to be persuaded that the system will not result in an increase in finances, and parents and advocates that it is not a means of cutting budgets, despite the pilot findings denying both of those outcomes. Parents will also need to be convinced that they will not have the entire responsibility for managing their family member's lives thrown back on them, and that there is provision for those without families, or whose families are disinterested, despite the clear call for a network of brokers and agencies to deal with these sorts of issues, that caused problems with Direct Payments. Above all, the use of the FACS criteria to deny people access to *In Control*, by their needs being assessed in the lower categories, probably by LAs facing ever tighter budgets themselves, would mean that the whole point of this initiative, which is to enable people to live their lives in ways that they, and not service budgets, dictate, will be missed. Experience from other countries, as we have seen, show the dangers of individualized budgets being used as a form of lottery, with more losers than winners.

Beyond the concerns about services' capacity to deliver individualized budgets, however, which lead to the impression that Adam's life in England, were he a random person with Down's syndrome, would be very different to what is actually happening, a wider thought remains. This is not new, but is cast into a new light for me by the experience of the visits to other countries. It concerns the impossibility of services ever creating an 'ordinary life' for people who do not fit the increasingly consumerist definition of what is ordinary. As our relationships become as commodified as everything else, and the expectation of being able to buy happiness, along with everything else on the supermarket shelf (or second-hand on e-Bay), is taken in with mother's milk (or formula), where are we going to get the personal, unpaid commitment to people with intellectual disabilities that defends them against the assumption of worthlessness? Perhaps the final chapter can bring some sort of answer, as we end this one with the final impression of 'Adam back home'.

ADAM BACK HOME

An adult in England

To quote from the box on education, Adam's adult life would also vary 'with both the location and the class of us as parents, and how 'pushy' we were'. He would, unless we had an *In Control* project running in our area, and we knew about it, almost certainly go to college after leaving school, though if he had more severe impairments he might go straight to day services, probably in a day centre, though possibly to an NHS-funded service which combined residential and day care. If he did go to college, some attempts in some places might be made to get Adam work experience, again depending on the degree of our pushing and the ethos of the particular college. Otherwise Adam would stay at college for some years, depending on whether the government tightened up rules about having to complete qualifications and whether he would be able to keep switching courses. Once college was finished, or in combinations of different days between college and day services, Adam would be offered a varying amount of time in day services. The LA interpretation of the FACS criteria would determine whether he was offered anything at all, as would the degree to which we as parents were prepared to refuse to provide support. This would be especially true if we declared ourselves unable to support Adam at home, since however capable he was, simply casting him out on his own would be deemed a 'crisis'. What he would be offered in that case would depend again on where we lived, though it would also relate to Adam's needs for support, especially if he had severe physical impairments or 'challenging behaviour', when arguments might well be held between the LA and the local PCT of the NHS as to who should finance the service. If we did not throw Adam out, however, but were reliant on services, he would probably join the significant number of adults living at home with us, his parents. If we were more 'pushy', or relatively financially secure, then we could think about the possibility of Direct Payments for an independent living situation for Adam, or a more flexible individualized budget from *In Control* if it were operating in our area. Even if it were, Adam would have to be deemed eligible for services under the FACS criteria. As for a job, the presence of some form of supported employment scheme, especially one which also made use of Workstep, would be an option we could go for, though again our class and financial status might well affect chances of success.

At the age of 22, and as a pretty competent person with Down's syndrome, the most likely possibility for Adam in 2006 would still be that his days would be spent at a combination of day services and college, and that he would be living with us in the family home. What happened in his leisure time would then also be highly dependent on where we lived and who we were, rather more than on who Adam was, and what he might want for his life. The reality of Adam's actual life at present is a rare combination of circumstances that owes a great deal to fortune, though, as his favourite football manager would say 'quality players make their own luck' – Adam is certainly a quality player.

9   Last thoughts, hopes and fears

Thus grew the tale of Wonderland:
Thus slowly, one by one,
Its quaint events were hammered out –
And now the tale is done. . . .

Lay it where Childhood's dreams are twined
In Memory's mystic band,
Like pilgrim's wither'd wreath of flowers
Pluck'd in a far-off land.

(Lewis Carroll)

Introduction

This final chapter is in two parts. First, a summary, in the style of the Adam's World Tour boxes that have been used throughout, of Adam's and our, chances of different services in different parts of the world. A broader reflection follows, on the issues that appear to me to affect services in the seven countries, and the hopes and fears this generates for the future of people like Adam. The chapter, and the book, will close with a final personal reflection on the whole experience.

ADAM'S WORLD CHANCES

What are they? What would be different in the seven countries?

Adam would probably have a greater chance of being born in Sweden and Norway than elsewhere, if we as parents knew nothing about Down's syndrome and my wife

---

was not over 35. Regardless of our position and age, screening and pressure for abortion of disabled children are significant in all the different countries, and all bar those two seem to present a high chance of Adam being 'screened out' unless we were very determined that we would have a child regardless.

If he were born, we, as Adam's parents, would probably get a very similar amount of attention in all countries during the early few years of his life, though if we were poor parents in the USA, this might be questionable. Equally, if his intellectual disability were less obvious than Down's syndrome, then whether he got classified as such would probably depend a lot, in all countries except the Scandinavian ones, on our financial and social status. The extent of what we received, if he were so classified, would also vary with such statuses, as well as our precise geographical location, though we would probably get something, especially 'respite', if he had severe disabilities. Whether the assistance was in our home would be more variable, though most countries have some good 'shared care' schemes in certain locations. Pre-school education options, and then school education itself, would probably be very different for Adam in the different countries, and in different parts of those countries. In most other countries than, again, Scandinavia, especially the USA and Canada, our ability to press for things (and to pay) would have a considerable impact on the degree of inclusion we might achieve for Adam, as would the nature of our immediate community. The classification of need for people with less obvious intellectual disabilities appears to be highly variable, and for both this and any resultant services our exact geographic location, in the USA, Canada, Australia and England, would again be a significant factor. The likelihood of access to mainstream schools *without parental pressure* (i.e. if we took what we were given) also appears to be very variable within the non-Scandinavian countries, though for different reasons, some to do with regional government policies, some local school board decisions. In Sweden and Norway the chances of inclusion regardless of parental influence are good, though people with severe disabilities in Sweden will normally go to separate schools. If Adam were on the autistic spectrum, there would be many more difficulties in all the countries. Given that there usually is parental pressure, and also because there are more supports for parental advocacy, mainstream inclusion in Canada, the USA, Australia and New Zealand, though variable, still appears more likely than England, but to be more often in 'units' once secondary school age has been reached.

Adam would be likely, if he were in mainstream schooling, to undertake a curriculum related to work in his teenage years at school in all countries other than England, where he would go up to 16 with much more emphasis on the academic syllabus and national examinations. He would also do some work-related things in the special schools in England, though there are less of these in most of the other countries. In those other countries, more people appear to stay on at school to 19–21, with a move to sheltered work or day services (or nothing, still a significant probability, especially in Australia) coming straight from school. In England, on the other hand, the route out of school is largely to college, with a few people going straight to adult day services.

Possibilities of open employment, in the full sense of that word, are fairly rare in all the countries, but meaningful daytime occupation, of a work-like nature, seems more prevalent in Sweden, Norway, Australia and New Zealand, with Australia achieving some level of payment and conditions close to open employment in some of its sheltered workshops. Despite some highly radical examples in the USA and Canada, and a slightly higher level of real employment, Adam would still be more likely to be in a sheltered workshop in both those countries. In all countries except the Scandinavian pair, if he were more disabled, or had behavioural problems, then there would also be a chance of Adam being in an institution during the daytime, which leads on to the possibilities for where he might live as an adult.

Getting a place of his own, and with whom he chooses to live, is again much more likely in Sweden and Norway. Though the other countries have some excellent residential services, they also have issues of access to those services, and the presence of many more institutional living situations, whether formally defined as such (as in 'over 16 people' in the USA) or as they would be defined by SRV (segregated and/or congregated places with groups of people living together who have not chosen to be with the others). Adam would probably have a greater choice, of who he lived with and where he lived, if he were in the relatively few radical projects in all the non-Scandinavian countries, but there would be a far higher probability, if he were the competent person with Down's syndrome that he is, that he would still be living in the family home with us.

As Adam's parents, we would need to be much more active in the USA than any other country, but still strongly so in England, Canada, Australia and New Zealand if we were to achieve anything beyond a very basic level of service (or anything at all). If we were not active, for whatever reason, we would probably get a far closer approximation to a life for Adam that accorded with SRV (or normalization in Sweden) if he lived in the Scandinavian countries. On the other hand, if we were active and committed to SRV ideas, there would be some chances in all the other countries of achieving an even closer fit to the 'good things of life' for Adam. For all of the non-Scandinavian group as well, however, especially the USA, Canada, England and Australia, it would be a significant advantage if we had money, as the chances of us being offered what we, and Adam, might think was a good life without some payment appear to be much less in those countries.

As for Adam getting what he has got – namely, a job; a day service that has meaning for him (though less valued by others); a house of his own shared with someone he wants to be with, independent of us, his parents, but still near enough for us to be of support; and in a village where he has a number of valued roles – then a great many rolls of a great many dice need to come up with sixes. Still more for him to add what he would probably regard as the greatest prize that he *hasn't* got, namely a really close personal relationship. The low odds, of course, of Adam achieving even as much as he has done would hold good in all countries, but they might be a little less stacked in Norway and Sweden. There, in my view, a higher number of people get close to more 'ordinary lives'. In the other countries there are shining examples of people who get even closer than Adam to the 'good life', but, like the Disneyland parade, they shine because of their rarity, and distract from the cardboard facade of the rest of Main Street.

Hopes and fears – influences on intellectual disability services

Figure 9.1 is adapted from a schema I used in a book on 'community care' in the UK (Malin et al. 1999). It tried to give a sense of the interaction of wider forces with those peculiar to intellectual disabilities, and is a series of inter-acting oval shapes, each representing elements that impact on services, but on each other as well. Most of the connecting arrows are two-way, with only the political ideology of the government leading to laws and funding having a one-way arrow. There is no attempt to suggest any sort of 'weighting' to the different influences, and we have seen how, in a number of specific instances in the different countries, what was an important influence at a particular point in time and in a particular place has much less effect somewhere else or

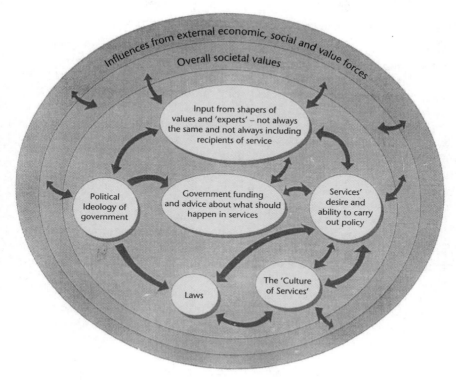

Figure 9.1 Influences on intellectual disability services

at some other time. So not only is this diagram meant to represent the fluidity of these forces, it is also trying to convey the complexity and dynamic nature of the service systems. Note, too, that little mention of people with intellectual disabilities and their families is contained in the diagram, except as the 'recipients of services' whose expertise is not always included in the 'input from shapers of values and experts'. This is also deliberate, since the schema is trying to look at forces which shape the *service system*, not the production of particular services for an individual. Of course, the system then impacts on individuals, in ways we have seen, and some of the individualized funding initiatives we have discussed could be said to be a way of replacing the system with individually organized support for ordinary lives. Even here, however, the system as a whole has to commit to at least funding the individual's freedom from it, or control over aspects of it, and that commitment, I would suggest, is greatly affected by the interaction of these same forces.

Influences from external economic, social and value forces

We have considered, at various points, the effects on services of the worldwide phenomena of the neo-liberal agenda and its offshoot, managerialism (Raper 2000; DiNitto and Cummins 2004), at least in the industrialized world. The main effects we saw realized in the non-Scandinavian countries, where they have created (or perpetuated in the case of the USA) either a real or a 'quasi-market' (Le Grand and Bartlett 1993) of welfare. Even in Norway and Sweden, however, although the managerialism element seems less, with professional dominance and legal requirements more powerful than economic determinants of amounts given to welfare and how services are governed, moves towards a market-based approach have been noticed by commentators (Harrison and Calltorp 2000; Waerness 2005). The picture hinted at by the relative welfare spending figures in Chapter 1 seems, therefore, to be supported by the detail of the countries' services, with pressure being felt far more from the global forces towards market-based welfare than those defending a universalist welfare state. Even some of the moves towards individualized funding, welcome from many perspectives as offering greater choice for service recipients and families, can be seen as a reflection of global moves towards consumerism. Certainly dressed in the language of 'choice and control' that goes with consumerism, the downside to such initiatives is that where *no* funding is allocated at all, or very little, then being able to spend the funding as one wishes has very little meaning.

Two other global forces that seem to affect the lives of people with intellectual disabilities, and therefore services to support them, are the growth of what has been called the 'knowledge economy' (Giddens 1990) and its awkward values bedfellow, postmodernism. The latter philosophical position, essentially rejecting the claim that there is such a thing as objective knowledge (Butler 2002), still sits uneasily with a world, and a service world, strongly based on assumptions that scientific and technological knowledge can deal with all human problems (Landes 2003). Neither view, of course, holds absolute sway, and though postmodernism can counter some of the positivist assertions regarding intellectual disability that were at the root of eugenic movements in all the countries, it does not seem to have prevented *de facto* eugenics through genetic screening and selective abortion from being the dominant picture in all the countries. Indeed, the 'knowledge' on which such practices are based has become to a great extent 'accepted wisdom' in many countries, namely that it is a 'tragedy' to have a child such as Adam, and that he (and of course more importantly in this individualist age, we) would be better off were he not born. On the other hand, however, the development of the 'knowledge economy' and much greater worldwide communication, has meant that such a version of reality can be challenged by stories of real people reaching a wider audience.

Postmodernism has also had the effect of lowering respect for, and raising doubts about, societal institutions such as health and education systems, which previously stood firm even when the more obvious flaws of the physical institutions in the different countries were revealed, especially by normalization. There appears now to be much more of a free for all, which of course fits in with the neo-liberal agenda, and also applies to values positions. We noted the role of Christianity in all the early services in our countries, but given that the place of religion, as another societal institution, has also been subject to the effects of postmodernism, on top of its previous pounding from scientific modernism, the values deriving from Judaeo-Christianity have also taken their place in the postmodern soup (Lyon 2000).

All of which means, in my view, that the dilution of a more agreed position on values relating to services, though that position had definite good and bad news about it, has led to the influence on services of a coherent values-based approach such as normalization/SRV being similarly diluted. It also means that the increased emphasis in postmodernism on image over substance enables many service systems, and even government strategies, to present themselves as adhering to a particular values position, without the need to let that values position outweigh the requirements of the market. Genuinely values-led and radical services then have to stand alongside the 'loss leaders' of the welfare market, and find their own 'niche', without being the major challenge to the status quo that they once were. Again this is less true in Scandinavia, where the greater specificity of the law and the lack of a market ensure consistency, sometimes at the expense of creativity, which of course is always the neo-liberal argument against state provision.

Finally, on a more practical level, the 'knowledge economy' with its increasing need for technological and social, as well as basic, literacy, can be seen as a major influence keeping people with intellectual disabilities in a dependent position. Struggling to read and write, even to talk, has not played well in industrialized societies for at least the last century. Not being able to use a computer or mobile telephone, to remember passwords and pin numbers, or to have a 'good telephone manner', all more likely for people with intellectual disabilities, not only affects their chances of employment, but also simply living in modern society.

Overall societal values

In keeping with the fluid nature of the schema, we have already begun to look at differences between the societies in terms of values, by noting their fairly consistent response to the postmodern globalized economy. The least affected, in my view, Norway and Sweden, owe that to the maintenance of a values position *vis-à-vis* the state provision of welfare. The fact that such a values position coincides with the state provision of intellectual disability services reflecting, or at least deriving from, a normalization/SRV perspective, is some-thing I would regard as positive. I would go further, however, and suggest, as I did in the respective chapters, that the nature of those two societies, at the values level, facilitates adherence to a *citizenship*, rather than a *deficit* model regarding intellectual disability (Armstrong and Barton 1999). At a lecture recently given to my UK students by a colleague from Sweden, much of the questioning was on her unspoken values assumption that it was 'right' for the state to provide support services to its citizens, regardless of disability or, importantly, the social and economic status of people and their families. Understanding of this basic value would, I believe, have been much more readily achieved with a group of English students when I first started in this field, and would have been shared by many more people in English society than is the case with 'Thatcher's children'. Of course, it is arguable whether Thatcher merely released an underlying competitive and class-envious society from the artificial shackles of the post-war welfare state, or created an entirely new generation in her own image, but the result seems the same, in that my students, all thoroughly committed to the welfare of people with intellectual disabilities, could not see how economics and power entered into the provi-sion of services in such a different way in Sweden. My impression of the overall values position of the other countries of this book was that they ranged from somewhere near the English position (old welfare state – now more and more market-driven) to somewhere close to the USA (always market-driven, but with such local variation that the impact of the market is equally variable). I would put New Zealand nearest to England in terms of the basic assumption of support being funded by the state, but, like Australia and Canada, moving towards the US position in terms of provision coming from the market. The influence of religious, specifically Christian, values on Swedish and Norwegian society, though without the state religion experience of England, again seemed to have an effect on services, but in broad terms and allied with the socialist position of the government. The effects of Judaeo-Christian values on the other societies appeared less in overall terms, with the exception of the USA, though highly important for specific services and agencies in all countries. In the USA, the place of religion is significant, but as part of the totally complex web of beliefs and values that permeate that society. In terms of services, this also means that the value bases of services can also accommodate a whole range, making it impossible to generalize, leaving the USA as a country that appears to contain, in terms of values, the most radical services and the most reactionary.

Input from shapers of values and 'experts'

Once again, the outer two influences in Figure 9.1 affect, and are affected by, those on the inside, not least in terms of what is considered 'expertise' in any particular area. One of the interesting things about working in intellectual disability for 30 years, but not entering the field through a professional route, is that one can observe the changing power of the different professional 'camps' over that period. In England, from an academic perspective, intellectual disability has remained a very small pool beyond which even the largest fish are not often allowed to venture. Dominated up to the 1960s by psychiatrists, who still remain in some positions of authority, the 1970s and 1980s saw the rise of the psychologists, who to date retain that dominance, especially the behaviourists. The normalization movement did not include many academics, one of the reasons perhaps it faced an academic backlash in the late 1980s, and since its decline as a force in England, that position has been maintained. In fact, though a number of the research units of the 1970s did have some effect; changes in *practice* in services in the last two decades of the twentieth century seem to have been far more influenced by PASS and PASSING workshops than by academic publications (Race 1999). So the 'shapers of values and experts' in England have, I believe, been found within the service world itself. A question I asked a number of people on my trip was 'Who would fill a conference of practitioners/parents?' and 'Who would fill a conference of academics?' My answer to these questions for England would be 'nobody' for the second question, and a couple of names, either from practice or practice 'consultants', for the first, all of whom would have had some connection with the normalization/SRV movement, even though some might now deny those origins. The answer I got in the different countries was similar in many respects, though most people added a rider, which I would have done, that the situation would have been very different 20 years ago. This latter point shows the effect, I believe, of postmodernism, in that the very notion of an 'expert' has been significantly challenged, and it also leads to the much more frequent response of my informants – namely that if the conference was headed up by people with intellectual disabilities, regardless of individuals, then a good turn-out would be likely from the practitioners and parents. Variation between countries on this followed familiar lines. Certain academics in Sweden and Norway, especially members of their own network, the NNDR, would generate a strong conference attendance, but for most of the other countries, the global forces on academia tended to produce the response that, like Disneyland, it was more important to go to events than what you heard or did there, and as for their proceedings, or much else in academic output, having any effect on services, the illusion was rather greater than the reality (a fact I must bear with in my hopes for this book). So the very forces that have produced a supermarket of services have produced a supermarket of experts, and they seem to stick with their own kind. Given what I also discovered, that specialized professional training in intellectual disability, especially at degree level, outside of England was somewhat rare, then what informs services in terms of the input from 'experts' during professional training is usually only as part of a more generic professional programme. The English maintenance of a specialist nursing qualification in intellectual disability, part of the continuing divide between the NHS and LAs, was met with amusement and ridicule in many countries, though the more thoughtful of my discussants did reflect on the problems in their countries in dealing with the health needs of people. Otherwise, the influences of shapers of values and experts in the different countries seemed to be strongly connected to the particular agency or sort of services I was talking to and about, with the inevitable bias, given my networks, towards SRV/normalization. Overall, therefore, the experience we had with Adam's PATH session, noted in Chapter 8, of a worldwide expert being totally unknown to all of the service people present, would seem to be the reality. Of far more immediate impact to most service-based people was the next element in our schema.

Government funding and advice about what should happen in services

Beyond the simple 'level of resources', so beloved of service systems as reasons for inaction or cuts, the *detail* of government funding, and the variation between the countries in terms of the *level* of government from which both funding and advice comes, seem to me to have a significant effect on services. The relative power of State and Provincial governments in Australia, Canada, and the USA, especially the latter two, make one's specific geographical location far more important in those countries. The CSTDA in Australia adds a further dimension to this, with the split between the funding of certain services by central government and the STs creating both opportunities and grave threats to people in that country, in the sense that the two sources can offer two chances of funding, but also a gap between which parents can fall. The autonomy of States and Provinces in the USA and Canada means that national initiatives appear to have less immediate effect than regional government policies, though the use of national funding streams in the USA appears to be important in States' service provision. The key point here appears to be who *controls* how the majority of the funding is spent, and in both the USA and Canada, this is clearly below central government level. Having a *national* policy which must be applied locally, as in New Zealand, Sweden and Norway, then presents different issues. If the national policy is also backed up by law, as in Scandinavia, as well as being administered and provided by local government, then consistency across the country is much more likely. New Zealand's agency-based approach, where both the commissioning and provision of services are theoretically independent, means that the variation is not geographical in the sense of local government having a significant impact, but more between the agencies, with the dominant power of IHC producing an important slant to the picture. All those three countries, however, together with England, do at least have a national set of policies that can act as a benchmark for services, though that of New Zealand and England is rather less specific than that of Scandinavia. In addition, the application of *de facto* rationing criteria at national level, as in the FACS policy in England, means that central government still has a significant impact on who gets services at all, which in turn relates to national finances beyond the specific intellectual disability field. The further complication, in England, of a centrally controlled NHS, but a partially centrally controlled (through finance) Local Authority both being commissioners of services, and also having a part to play in provision, only adds to the variation in influence of governments at national and local level. What drives that funding and advice, as Figure 9.1 shows, is affected by the political ideology of the government, and whether it uses laws to attempt to get things achieved. These two elements will be taken together.

Political ideology of government and use of laws

As before, the interactions between our elements are perhaps more important than the elements themselves. The variation we have noted above in the power of the different levels of government means that the political ideology at each level becomes more or less important. In the Scandinavian countries, the long reign of socialist governments has clearly contributed to the maintenance of the welfare states, and the overall societal values of citizenship of those countries seems to generate an assumption that government policies and laws are there for the good of the people of the country. Whether this is true in reality, it certainly appears to be the case that prescriptive laws on services are accepted and acted on as the guides and standards by which services must operate, and to which the local government bodies are held accountable. The political ideology of the New Labour government in England, however, even though different from its predecessor (not as much as some socialists would like) does not seem to have brought about a significant change in how services are organized or financed. This may be because the moves of Thatcherism to dismantle the welfare state, based on the neo-liberal ideology also displayed by governments in the USA, Australia, and earlier in New Zealand, did not quite succeed, but left the totally confusing mixture of a quasi-market in welfare that we still have. The market-driven ideology, of course, does not like government intervention, least of all in formal laws, and it is no surprise that in the non-Scandinavian countries there are very few *specific* laws that determine practice. If we add in the power of States and Provinces in Australia, Canada and the USA to make their own laws, then the impact of *statute* law on intellectual disability services in all the non-Scandinavian countries is extremely variable, both within and between the countries. All have some form of anti-discrimination legislation, and this has been an important protection for people with intellectual disabilities, as well as leading to some important *case law* judgments, especially in the USA, though again regional and local variation in judicial powers and types of action means generalization is impossible.

Overall, therefore, the political ideology of governments could be said to have had a significant impact on services in general, with the obvious contrasts between the more socialist-oriented Scandinavians, the very mixed bag that is New Labour in England, the various coalitions in New Zealand that followed from electoral reform, and then the neo-liberal regimes at national level in Australia and the USA, recently joined by Canada, who already had such regimes at the Provincial level, as did the USA. On intellectual disability services specifically, however, the influence of political ideology is probably much less significant, with the use of laws somewhat scarce. This leaves us the last two of our elements, which will again be taken together.

Services' desire and ability to carry out policy – the 'culture of services'

Above all other elements, in my view, these two represent the greatest influences on the actual lives of service recipients and yet are themselves the most affected by the wider influences. By this I mean that what people actually receive is most powerfully affected by the services' desire and ability to carry out policy, but the nature and clarity of what policies mean, and the resources to put them into effect, can, on the one hand, create a 'culture' of services in accord with the policy, but on the other, a culture of resistance to change, preservation of jobs and existing forms of service, which makes the impact of policies virtually nil. We have already seen, looking at the other elements of our schema, how much more varied their effects are in the non-Scandinavian countries, so we will begin with Norway and Sweden as the most straightforward. My impression in this regard is that, given the long history of welfare states in those two countries, the power of national policies and laws, the degree of qualification of staff, and the national monitoring of standards, most services respond to policies with a sense of professionalism and commitment to a commonly agreed set of values. The 'culture' of services in both countries therefore appeared to me to be one which held good across the country as a whole, with a level of service delivery consistently in accord with the notions of normalization/SRV, though probably more the former than the latter, especially in Sweden. This does not, of course, mean they are beyond criticism, and conformity to standards has some effects that would be considered less than satisfactory in certain parts of the other countries, for example, the segregated 'training schools' for severely disabled children in Sweden, or the limited open employment possibilities in both countries.

Overall, however, the interaction of the various forces in our schema seems to me to have produced, to date, a fairly consistent level of service across these two countries, with only threats to the overall welfare state likely to upset that balance.

All the other countries, in my view, show a much greater tension between the various elements, combined with an inconsistency across the different parts of the countries that makes it almost impossible to speak of a single response to the questions of services' desire and ability to carry out policy, or of their 'culture'. This is partly a weakness of the schema, in that its origins in the much more uniform English welfare state of two decades ago, when England was much closer to Scandinavia in service structures, if not actual services, lends itself to the notion of an overall pattern. Equally, though, the fact of tensions between individual services and service agencies' desires to carry out particular policies, and the funding constraints that flow from national and international trends in ideology and market forces illustrates how variable services are on the ground in the individual countries. In England and New Zealand, what appear to be positive national strategies can be, and are being, undone or hindered both by the funding constraints of 'prudent' governments, but also by the different value positions of the different agencies and professional groupings competing for those funds. Developing a 'culture' in agencies to respond to the fairly radical value positions of *Valuing People* or the NZDS is inevitably at odds with the constraints of a welfare market, though such a market does provide 'niches' for some really excellent and creative things to develop.

There also seems to be a difference in the degree of uniformity between children's services, including schools, and services for adults, in all the non-Scandinavian countries. The ethos of publicly provided education, and early childhood support, perhaps because it has a greater genericism than services for adults, but also because of the influence of broader values positions, seems to me to provide a greater chance of at least some services being provided to all children. In the case of education, the notion of inclusion seems to have at least gained a substantial foothold in the service culture. Given also that government funding in all countries tends to be focused on children, the possibility of broad policies such as inclusion being at least significantly followed is that much greater.

When it comes to adult services, however, the degree of variation noted above in New Zealand and England is magnified in the other three countries, in my view. This is not just to do with the greater power of regional governments, though that is certainly significant, nor with the neo-liberal ideology of, especially, Australia and much of the USA, but the combination of those forces, input from a whole range of 'shapers of values and experts', including, but far from only, promoters of SRV and the social model of disability, and the basic competitive organizational struggle for existence of agencies. Agencies

with the desire to carry out radical policies may face local or national governments with no commitment to such policies, thus emasculating the agencies'
ability to carry them out; those with a more market-oriented agenda may find
ways round more radical government policies, relying on the vagueness of
practical specification and the inevitable rationing to make a case for their
services. Their culture becomes that of business organizations, with pressure
on their values positions from the basic organizational values of survival and
expansion. Hence the constant repetition of the phrase, in Australia, Canada
and the USA in particular, but also England and New Zealand, that 'it depends
where you live'. There are many examples in all those countries of services
and agencies whose 'culture' is all about supporting people with intellectual
disabilities to find valued lives in their communities, but there are equally
many, if not more, where this culture is tinged by, or even taken over by,
cultures of organizational loyalty and promotion, bureaucratic box-ticking, or
professional corner defending.

What this produces, of course, is the huge range of services and
organizational arrangements that this book has struggled to describe. We
close, however, with a personal reflection, not from 'the data' but from
the gut.

A final reflection – people, not services, lead ordinary lives

An English historian, Professor Geoffrey Hosking, addressing the Royal Historical Society in 2004 as part of a seminar entitled 'Can we construct a history of
trust?' pondered on what he saw as a phenomenon of Western cultures, the
replacement of faith in political and social judgements by mere quantification
of money. He went on to talk about this in the English context, with reference
to the earlier trust in public institutions being partly a reflection of deference
within the class system, exposed as dubious by greater information and education of the 'lower classes' in the twentieth century, especially its latter half.
Instead of an informed public holding public institutions to account, however,
the 'emperor's new clothes' phenomenon had generated a 'blame and shame'
culture, especially of politicians, educators, lawyers, clergy, and even royalty,
and a belief that everything can be reduced to cash compensation. This then
created a 'vicious circle' where the public institutions then responded to the
culture, reinforcing its perceptions of their motivations. 'The more we place
our trust in institutions whose *raison d'être* is monetary operations, the more
we reshape our social lives according to the standards set by those operations'
(Hosking 2004: 5).

Apart from the similarity to the SRV notion of 'role circularity' in Hosking's
argument, my point in quoting him is to give academic support to my intense

feelings regarding the change in my society in the 30 years since I became involved in intellectual disability, and thus in the society into which we have tried to support Adam to become 'included'. That the change in the culture in that period has been led, from a media perspective, by an Australian, and by a government committed to an aping of the USA in a great many aspects of life, only makes the feeling more visceral. The world in which all my sons are 'included' seems a far scarier place than when I went, as a naïve researcher, to Reading University in 1973. My visits to the six countries did little to make my fears for them any the less, though the Scandinavian experience reminded me that some countries were still holding out against the globalizing tide, if with increasing difficulty.

Yet what I was left with, both on my return home and then at the end of the England chapter, was a different emotion, that of being part of a community, in which Adam had many valued roles, and I guess this is the essential issue that this book has revealed. Institutions, be they the vast snake-pits of the first half of the twentieth century suffered by people with intellectual disabilities, or the monarchy that still rules over half the countries I visited, exist because they serve societal purposes, often lost in the mists of time, and no longer logical, but still there. Ordinary lives, at the really local level, with all their variation, exist and are developed because they are about people making the best of who and what they are, and how they interact with each other. What societies can provide in terms of services for people with intellectual disabilities has a limit, which is that, however 'values-led' they may be, they are an artificial replacement for a family and a community. Therein lie both my hopes and fears. The increasing alienation of societies, especially in urban areas, where as we saw a large proportion of the population of the countries of this book live, and the reduction of so many human interactions to a commodity to be bought and sold, tends to push families and communities into their bunkers, afraid to 'risk' communication on an open basis, preferring the arm's length 'business basis'. 'Objective professional distance' could be said to be an art of both the social worker and the prostitute, though with more illusion of caring from the latter, and the more 'businesslike' the transaction is, the less exposure to vulnerability, possibly at the heart of real relationship, there will be.

The fact that, in the great majority of good things I saw or heard about, there would be a committed person, or group of people, or small community, often including parents and family members, tells me there is an underlying human characteristic that has not yet been ground down by the commodification of human experiences. Where services, in the organized sense, have allied themselves to this characteristic, they have, in my view, both set themselves up against the tide of the 'social approaches' of most countries, but also increased the hope I have that Adam's experiences need not be as hard to find on his world tour as they appeared to be. In the end, as the Màori saying has it:

He aha te mea nui?
He aha te mea nui o tea o?
Maku e ki atu.
He tangata. He tangata. He tangata.

What is the most important thing?
What is the most important thing in the world?
I will say to you.
It is people. It is people. It is people.

Bibliography

access ability (2003) *Report to the Ministry of Health: Overview of Residential Service Provision for People with an Intellectual Disability within Auckland*. Auckland: access ability.

Aday, L.A. (2001) *At Risk in America: The Health and Health Care Needs of Vulnerable Populations in the United States*, 2nd edn. Hoboken, NJ: Jossey-Bass.

Alaszewski, A. (1986) *Institutional Care and the Mentally Handicapped*. London: Croom Helm.

Alcock, P. and Craig, G. (eds) (2001) *International Social Policy: Welfare Regimes in the Developed World*. Basingstoke: Palgrave Macmillan.

Allen, T.F., Traustadottir, R. and Spina, L. (2005) 'In the Community' and 'A New Life' in K. Johnson, and R. Traustadottir (eds) *Deinstitutionalization and People with Intellectual Disabilities*. London: Jessica Kingsley Publishers.

Andrews, J. and Lupart, J. (2000) *The Inclusive Classroom: Educating Exceptional Children*. Scarborough, Ontario: Nelson, Thompson Learning.

Anisef, P. and Lanphier, M. (eds) (2003) *The World is a City*. Toronto: University of Toronto Press.

Annerén, G. and Ollars, B. (2004) Sweden, in P. Boyd, C. de Vigan and E. Garne (eds) *Special Report: Pre-natal Screening Policies in Europe*. Newtownabbey, County Antrim: University of Ulster.

Argent, H. and Kerrane, A. (1997) *Taking Extra Care: Respite, Shared and Permanent Care for Children with Disabilities* London: British Agencies for Adoption and Fostering (BAAF).

Armstrong, F. and Barton, L. (eds) (1999) *Disability, Human Rights and Education*. Buckingham: Open University Press.

Asch, A. (1999) Pre-natal diagnosis and selective abortion: a challenge to practice and policy, *American Journal of Public Health*, 89(11): 1649–57.

Australian Healthcare Associates (2005) *Commonwealth State/Territory Disability Agreement Annual Public Report 2003–04*. Canberra: Australian Government Department of Family and Community Services.

Australian Institute of Health and Welfare (AIHW) (2005) *Disability Support Services 2003–2004: National Data on Services Provided under the Commonwealth State/Territory Disability Agreement*. Canberra: AIHW.

Bach, M. (2002) Social inclusion as solidarity: rethinking the Child Rights Agenda, in *Perspectives in Social Inclusion: Summaries*. Occasional Papers Series No 3. Toronto: The Laidlaw Foundation.

Bagnell, K. (1980) *The Little Immigrants*. Toronto: Macmillan.

Baldock, J., Manning, N. and Vickerstaff, S. (eds) (2003) *Social Policy*, 2nd edn. Oxford: Oxford University Press.

Ballard, K. (ed.) (1994) *Disability, Family, Whànau and Society*. Palmerston North: Dunmore Press.

Baranjay, E.P. (1971) *The Mentally Handicapped Adolescent*. Oxford: Pergamon.

Barnes, C., Mercer, G. and Shakespeare, T. (1999) *Exploring Disability: A Sociological Introduction*. Cambridge: Polity Press.

Barnes, C., Oliver, M. and Barton, L. (eds) (2002) *Disability Studies Today*. Cambridge: Polity Press.

Bartlett, W., Roberts, J. and Le Grand, J. (eds) (1998) *A Revolution in Social Policy: Quasi-market Reforms in the 1990s*. Bristol: Policy Press.

Barwick, H. (ed.) (2002) *Special Education 2000: Monitoring and Evaluation of the Policy – Final Report (Phase Three)*. New Zealand: Massey University.

Bean, P. and Melville, J. (1983) *Lost Children of the Empire*. London: Unwin Hyman.

Biklen, D., Kluth, P. and Straut, D. (eds) (2003) *Access to Academics for All Students: Critical Approaches to Inclusive Curriculum, Instruction, and Policy*. Mahweh, NJ: Erlbaum.

Blanchet, A. (1999) The Impact of Normalization and Social Role Valorization in Canada, in R.J. Flynn and R.A. Lemay (eds) *A Quarter Century of Normalization and Social Role Valorization: Evolution and Impact*. Ottawa: University of Ottawa.

Booth, T. and Ainscow, M. (eds) (1998) *From Them to Us: International Study of Inclusion in Education*. London: Routledge.

Broberg, G. and Roll-Hansen, N. (2005) *Eugenics and the Welfare State: Sterilization Policy in Norway, Sweden, Denmark, and Finland*. Michigan: Michigan State University Press.

Broda, T. (2004) Services for persons with intellectual and developmental disabilities in Montreal: a nurse's perspective, *International Journal of Nursing in Intellectual and Developmental Disabilities*, 1(1):7.

Brogan, H. (2001) *The Penguin History of the USA*, 2nd edn. London: Penguin.

Brown, H. and Smith, H. (1992) *Normalisation: A Reader for the Nineties*. London: Routledge.

Brown, R. (2003) *Disability and Society: Challenges in the 21st Century*. ASSID.

Brunton, W. (2006) Gray, Theodore Grant 1884–1964. *Dictionary of New Zealand Biography*, updated 7 April 2006. http://www.dnzb.govt.nz/ (accessed 25/01/07).

Buell, M.K. and Brown, I. (1999) Lifestyles of adults with developmental disabilities in Ontario, in I. Brown and M. Percy (eds) *Developmental Disabilities in Toronto*, 1st edn. Toronto: Ontario Association for Developmental Disabilities.

Bunch, G. and Valeo, A. (1997) *Inclusion: Recent Research*. Toronto: Inclusion Press.

Butler, C. (2002) *Postmodernism: A Very Short Introduction*. Oxford: Oxford University Press.

Cabinet Office, Department of Works and Pensions, Department of Health,

Department for Education and Skills, Office of the Deputy Prime Minister (2005) *Improving the Life Chances of Disabled People*. London: Cabinet Office.

Canadian Association for Community Living (CACL) (2005) *From Values to Action: Building a Community Living Movement for a Decade of Change*. Toronto: CACL.

Canadian Encyclopaedia (2007) *Social Gospel* http://www. canadianencyclopedia. ca/index.cfm?PgNm=TCE&Params=A1ARTA0007522 (accessed 27/01/07).

Canadian Mental Health Association (2006) *Our History*. http://www.cmha.ca/bins/ content_page.asp?cid=7–135 (accessed 27/11/06).

Capie, A. (1997) Evaluating human service delivery, in P. O'Brien and R. Murray (eds) *Human Services: Towards Partnership and Support*. Palmerston North: The Dunmore Press Ltd.

Carey, H.E. (1960) *The History of the New Zealand Crippled Children Society's First Twenty-five Years, 1935–1960*. Wellington: CCS.

Carling-Burzacott, R. (2004) *Disability as a Liberation Struggle and a New Rights Movement in Australia*. http://acqol.deakin.edu.au/Conferences/abstracts_pa-pers/2004/Carling.doc (accessed 26/01/07).

Carlson, C. (2000) *Involving All Neighbours: Building Inclusive Communities in Seattle*. Seattle: Department of Neighbourhoods.

Carvel, J. (2006) Time to make the figures add up, *The Guardian*, 12 April.

Castles, F., Gerritsen, R. and Vowels, J. (eds) (1996) *The Great Experiment: Labour Parties and Public Policy Transformation in Australia and New Zealand*. Auckland: Auckland University Press.

Castles, F. and Shirley, I. (1996) Labour and Social Policy: Gravediggers or Refur-bishers of the Welfare State, in F. Castles, R. Gerritsen and J. Vowels (eds) *The Great Experiment: Labour Parties and Public Policy Transformation in Australia and New Zealand*. Auckland: Auckland University Press.

Center for Reproductive Rights (2005) *The World's Abortion Laws*. http://www. crlp.org/pub_fac_abortion_laws.html (accessed 25/01/07).

Chaison, G.N. (2005) *Unions in America*. Thousand Oaks, CA: Sage Publications Inc.

Chappell, A.L. (1998) Still out in the cold, people with learning difficulties and the social model of disability, in T. Shakespeare (ed.) *The Disability Reader*. London: Cassell.

Chenoweth, L. (2000) Closing the doors: insights and reflections on deinsti-tutionalisation. *Law in Context*, 17(2): 77–100.

Cheyne, C., O'Brien, M. and Belgrave, M. (2000) *Social Policy in Aotearoa New Zealand: A Critical Introduction*, 2nd edn. Auckland: Oxford University Press.

Chupik, J. (2004) *The Institutional Confinement of 'Idiot' Children in Twentieth-century Canada: The Case of the Orillia Asylum, 1900–1950*. http://www.shermandorn. com/hec/archives/000142.html#more (accessed 18/11/06).

Churchill, W.S. (1909) *Liberalism and the Social Problem*. London: Hodder & Stoughton.

Clarke, J., Gewirtz, S. and McLaughlin, E. (eds) (2000) *New Managerialism, New Welfare*. London: Sage Publications Ltd.

Clarke, P. (1998) The Rise and Fall of Thatcherism, *London Review of Books* 20(2).

Cocks, E. (2005) *International issues and trends in disability services*. Presentation to the ACROD Chief Executive Officers Conference, Canberra, 23–24 November 2005.

Cocks, E., Fox, C., Brogan, M. and Lee, M. (eds) (1996) *Under Blue Skies: The Social Construction of Intellectual Disability in Western Australia*. Perth: Edith Cowan University.

Cohen, A., Butterworth, J., Gilmore, D. and Metzel, D. (2003) *High Performing States in Integrated Employment* (Research to Practice 9(1)). Boston, MA: University of Massachusetts, Boston, Institute for Community Inclusion.

Coleman, J.C. (1988) Social capital in the creation of human capital, *American Journal of Sociology*, 94: S95-S120.

Community Resource Unit (CRU) (2003) *Relationships and Everyday Lives*. Brisbane: CRU.

Community Resource Unit (CRU) (2005) *The Challenge of Inclusion: People Labelled with 'Challenging Behaviour' and the Struggle to Belong*. Conference Papers 2005. Brisbane: CRU.

Community Resource Unit (CRU) (2007) website http://www.cru.org.au/ (accessed 27/01/07).

Cox, C. and Pearson, M. (1995) *Made to Care: The Case for Residential and Village Communities for People with a Mental Handicap*. Stockport: RESCARE.

Croft, D. (2000) *When Needs Go Begging*. West Perth: Developmental Disability Council of Western Australia (DDC).

Crook, D.R., Power, S. and Whitty, S. (1999) *The Grammar School Question*. London: Institute for Education.

Crossman, R. (1977) *The Diaries of a Cabinet Minister*, Vol. 3. London: Hamish Hamilton.

Cutler, T. and Waine, B. (1997) *Managing the Welfare State*. Oxford: Berg.

Daily Mail (2005) Immigrants make up half Britain's population growth, 7 September 2005. http://www.dailymail.co.uk/pages/live/articles/news/news.html?in_article_id=361617&in_page_id=1770

Davies, I. and Spencer, K. (2005) in E. Emerson, S. Malam, I. Davies and K. Spencer (eds) *Adults with Learning Disabilities in England 2003/04*. London: National Statistics and NHS Health and Social Care Information Centre.

Davis et al. v. California Health and Human Services Agency et al. (2003) http://www.bazelon.org/incourt/docket/Davis.html (accessed 30/01/07).

De Crespigny L.J. and Savulescu J. (2004) Abortion: time to clarify Australia's confusing laws. *Med J Aust*, 181: 201–3.

Department for Works and Pensions (DWP) (2005) *Opportunity Age: Meeting the Challenges of Aging in the 21st Century*. London: DWP.

Department of Education (DoE) (1988) *Tomorrow's Schools: The Reform of Education Administration in New Zealand*. Wellington: DoE.

Department of Education (DoE) (2003) *Enhancing Effective Practice in Special Education.* http://www.minedu.govt.nz/index.cfm?layout=document&documentid=9793&indexid=9825&indexparentid=7961 (accessed 26/01/07).

Department of Education (DoE) (2004) *Indicators of Effectiveness.* http://www.minedu.govt.nz/index.cfm?layout=document&documentid=10052&data=l (accessed 26/01/07).

Department of Education (DoE) (2006) *The Ongoing and Renewable Resources Schemes: Guidelines.* http://www.minedu.govt.nz/index.cfm?layout=document&documentid=5323&data=l (accessed 26/01/07).

Department of Disability, Housing and Community Services (DHCS) (2004) *Future Directions: A Framework for the ACT 2004–2008.* Canberra: DHCS.

Department of Health (DoH) (1988) *Community Care: Agenda for Action (The Griffiths Report).* London: HMSO.

Department of Health (DoH) (1989) *Caring for People: Community Care in the Next Decade and Beyond* (Cm 849). London: HMSO.

Department of Health (1999) *Facing the Facts: Services for People with Learning Disabilities: Policy Impact Study of Social Care and Health Services.* London: DoH.

Department of Health (2001) *Valuing People: A New Strategy for Learning Disability for the 21st century* (Cm 5086). London: The Stationery Office.

Department of Health (2003) *Fair Access to Care Services: Guidance on Eligibility Criteria for Adult Social Care.* London: DoH.

Department of Health (2005) *Independence, Well-Being and Choice: Our Vision for the Future of Social Care for Adults in England.* London: DoH.

Department of Health and Social Security (DHSS) (1971) *Better Services for the Mentally Handicapped.* (Cmd 4683). London: HMSO.

Derry, T.K. (1973) *A History of Modern Norway, 1814–1972.* Oxford: Oxford University Press.

Dileo, D. (2007) *Raymond's Room.* St Augustine, FL: Training Resource Network Inc.

DiNitto, D.M. and Cummins, L.K. (2004) *Social Welfare: Politics and Public Policy,* (Research Navigator Edition), 6th edn. Boston: Allyn and Bacon.

Disability Standards Review and Quality Assurance Working Party (1997) *Assuring Quality: A Report by the Disability Standards Review and Quality Assurance Working Party.* Canberra: Office of Disability.

Douglas, T. (1933) *The problems of the subnormal family.* MA thesis. Hamilton: McMaster University.

Durie, M. (2005) Race and ethnicity in public policy: does it work? *Social Policy Journal of New Zealand,* 24.

Emerson, E., Malam, S., Davies, I. and Spencer, K. (2005) *Adults with Learning Difficulties in England, 2003/2004.* London, National Statistics and NHS Health and Social Care Information Centre.

Emerson, E., Robertson, J., Gregory, N., Hatton, C., Kessisoglou, S. and Hallam, A. (1999) *Quality and Costs of Residential Supports for People with Learning*

Disabilities. Manchester: Hester Adrian Research Centre, University of Manchester.

Enteman, W.F. (1993) *Managerialism: The Emergence of a New Ideology*. Wisconsin: University of Wisconsin Press.

Ericsson, K. (1999) The shift between two traditions of support: Swedish experiences, in K. Ericsson (ed.) *Establishing CBR for Persons with Mental Retardation: A Task for the Swedish Integration Project in Amman*. Uppsala University, Department of Education, http://opus.uu.se/publication.xml?id=16381 (accessed 23/01/07).

Ericsson, K. (2000) *Deinstitutionalization and community living for persons with an intellectual disability in Sweden: policy, organizational change and personal consequences*. Presentation to Disability Conference, Tokyo.

Evang, K. (1955) *Sterilisering etter lov av 1. juni 1934 om adgang til sterilisering m.v.* Sarpsborg: F. Verding.

Falvey, M., Forest, M., Pearpoint, J. and Rosenberg, R. (1997) *All My Life's a Circle*. new expanded edition. Toronto: Inclusion Press.

Fennell, P. (1995) *Treatment Without Consent: Law, Psychiatry and the Treatment of Mentally Disordered People Since 1845*. London and New York: Routledge.

Fine, B. (2001) *Social Capital versus Social Theory: Political Economy and Social Science at the Turn of the Millennium*. London and New York: Routledge.

Flem, A., Moen, T. and Gudmundsdottir, S. (2004) Towards inclusive schools: a study of inclusive education in practice, *European Journal of Special Needs Education*, 19(1): 85–98.

Flynn, R.J. and Lemay, R.A. (eds) (1999) A *Quarter Century of Normalization and Social Role Valorization: Evolution and Impact*. Ottawa: University of Ottawa.

Flynn, R.J. and Nitsch, K.E. (1980) Normalization: accomplishments to date and future priorities, in R.J. Flynn and K.E. Nitsch (eds) *Normalization, Social Integration and Community Services*. Austin, TX: PRO-ED Inc.

Frazee, C. (2000) *Obscuring Disability: The Pursuit of Quality in the Canadian Biotechnology Strategy*. Toronto: National Network on Environments and Women's Health.

Freckleton, I. (2005) Institutional death: the coronial inquest into the deaths of nine men with intellectual disabilities, in K. Johnson, and R. Traustadottir (eds) *Deinstitutionalization and People with Intellectual Disabilities*. London & Philadelphia: Jessica Kingsley Publishers.

Freyhoff, G., Parker, C., Coue, M. and Greig, N. (eds) (2004) *Included in Society*. Brussels: Inclusion Europe.

FUB (1999) *FUB's Research Conference 10–11 June 1999: A Meeting between Researchers and People with Learning Disabilities*. Stockholm: FUB.

Giddens, A. (1990) *The Consequences of Modernity*. Cambridge: Polity Press.

Gilmore, D.S. and Butterworth, J. (1997) *Work Status Trends for People with Mental Retardation*. http://archives.communityinclusion.org/publications/text/rp3–97. html (accessed 30/01/07).

Gladwell, M. (2005) The moral-hazard myth, *The New Yorker*, 29 August.

Glasby, J. and Peck, E. (eds) (2004) *Care Trusts: Partnership Working in Action*. Abingdon: The Radcliffe Medical Press Ltd.

Goddard, H.H. (1912) *The Kallikak Family: A Study in the Heredity of Feeble Mindedness*. New York: Macmillan.

Goggin, G. and Newell, C. (2005) *Disability in Australia: Exposing a Social Apartheid*. Sydney: University of New South Wales Press Ltd.

Gould, A. (2001) *Developments in Swedish Social Policy*. Basingstoke: Palgrave Macmillan.

Gould, S.J. (1996) *The Mismeasure of Man*, 2nd edn. London: W. W. Norton & Co. Ltd.

Government Offices of Sweden (2007) http://www.sweden.gov.se/sb/d/2098 (accessed 23/01/07).

Gynnerstedt, K. (1997) Past, present and future for people with learning disabilities, *Journal of Learning Disabilities*, 1(3): 147–52.

Hadley, R. and Clough, R. (1996) *Care in Chaos: Frustration and Challenge in Community Care*. London: Cassell.

Handicapped Programs Review (Australia) (1985) *New Directions: Report of the Handicapped Programs Review*. Canberra: Australian Government Publishing Service.

Hansen, J. (2006) *Each Belongs: The Remarkable Story of the First School System to Move to Inclusion*. Toronto: Inclusion Press.

Harker, M. and King, N. (1999) *An Ordinary Home: Housing and Support for People with Learning Disabilities*. London: Local Government Association.

Harman A.D. (2006) *Investigating the Transition of Children with Autism from School, to the Community, Work, or Further Education*. http://www.assid.org.au/Portals/0/Downloads/Harman.pdf (accessed 27/01/06).

Harrington, M. (2004) *Commonwealth Funding for Schools Since 1996: An Update*. Research Note no. 41 2003–04. Canberra: Australia Parliamentary Library.

Harrison, M.I. and Calltorp, J. (2000) The re-orientation of market-oriented reforms in Swedish health care, *Health Policy*, 50: 219–40.

Hartnett, F. (1997) The challenges of living the practices of social valorization, in P. O'Brien and R. Murray (eds) *Human Services: Towards Partnership and Support*. Palmerston North: The Dunmore Press Ltd.

Haug, P. (2000) *Regimes of Special Education Research: Trends in special education research in Norway*. Paper presented at the European Research Association Conference, Edinburgh, 20–23 September.

Haug, P. (2004) *Inclusion in Norwegian Compulsory School*. Paper presented at the Nordic Educational Research Association Conference. Reykjavik, 11–13 March.

Hessle, S. and Vinnerljung, B. (1999) *Child Welfare in Sweden – An Overview*. Studies in Social Work No. 14, Stockholm: Department of Social Work, Stockholm University.

Hill, A. (2001) Social role valorization, *Clinical Psychology Forum*, 149: 9–12.

Hogan, M.F. (1980) Normalization and communitization, in R.J. Flynn and K.E. Nitsch (eds) *Normalization, Social Integration and Community Services*. Austin, TX: PRO-ED Inc.

Hollander, A. (1999) The origin of the Normalization principle in Sweden and its impact on legislation today, in R.J. Flynn and R.A. Lemay (eds) *A Quarter Century of Normalization and Social Role Valorization: Evolution and Impact*. Ottawa: University of Ottawa.

Holmes, J. and Wileman, T. (1995) *Toward Better Governance: Public Service Reform in New Zealand (1984–94) and its Relevance to Canada*. Ottawa: Office of the Auditor General of Canada. http://www.oag-bvg.gc.ca/domino/other.nsf/html /nzbody.html (accessed 25/01/07).

Homes West Association Inc. (HWAI) (2005) *Policies*. Sherwood: HWAI.

Hosking, G. (2004) *Why do we need a history of trust?* Paper presented to a Historical Society Study Day, 'Can we construct a history of trust?', 7 February.

Hudson, R. (1994) Management and finance, in N. Malin (ed.) *Implementing Community Care*. Buckingham: Open University Press.

Internet Modern History Sourcebook http://www.fordham.edu/halsall/mod/ modsbook28.html (accessed 23/01/07).

Irgens (2004) 'Norway' in P. Boyd, C. de Vigan and E. Garne (eds) (2005) *Prenatal Screening Policies in Europe* Special Report. Belfast: Univeristy of Ulster.

Jakobsen L.B., Moum, T. and Heiberg, A. (2000) Need of better knowledge of genetic tests among Norwegian physicians, *Tidsskr Nor Laegeforen*, 120(20): 2419–22.

Jay Committee (1979) *Report of the Committee of Inquiry into Mental Handicap Nursing and Care* (Cmd 7468). London: HMSO.

Johansen, E. and Kristiansen, K. (2005) Gone fishin: from institutional outing to real life, in K. Johnson, and R. Traustadottir (eds) *Deinstitutionalization and People with Intellectual Disabilities*. London & Philadelphia: Jessica Kingsley Publishers.

Johnson, K. (1998) *Deinstitutionalising Women: An Ethnographic Study of Institutional Closure*. Melbourne: Cambridge University Press.

Johnson, K. and Traustadottir, R. (eds) (2005) *Deinstitutionalization and People with Intellectual Disabilities*. London & Philadelphia: Jessica Kingsley Publishers.

Kautto, M., Heikkila, M., Hvinden, B., Marklund, S. and Ploug, N. (eds) (1999) *Nordic Social Policy*. London and New York: Routledge.

Key Indicators of the Labour Market (KILM) (2005) 4th edition http://www.ilo.org/ public/english/employment/strat/kilm/features.htm (accessed 30/01/07).

King's Fund (1984) *An Ordinary Working Life: Vocational Services for People with Mental Handicaps*. King's Fund Project Paper No. 50. London: King's Fund Centre.

Koomarri (2005) *Our Quality Journey*. Canberra: Koomarri Association ACT Inc.

Kristiansen, K. (1993) *Normalering og verdsetjing av social rolle*. Oslo: Kommune-forlaget.

Kristiansen, K. (1999) The impact of Normalization and Social Role Valorization in

Scandinavia, in R.J. Flynn and R.A. Lemay (eds) *A Quarter Century of Normalization and Social Role Valorization: Evolution and Impact*. Ottawa: University of Ottawa.

Kristiansen, K., Soder, M. and Tøssebro, J. (1999) Social integration in a welfare state: research from Norway and Sweden, in R.J. Flynn and R.A. Lemay (eds) *A Quarter Century of Normalization and Social Role Valorization: Evolution and Impact*. Ottawa: University of Ottawa.

Kugel, R. and Wolfensberger, W. (eds) (1969) *Changing Patterns in Residential Services for the Mentally Retarded*. Washington, DC: President's Committee on Mental Retardation, US Government Printing Office.

Laird, W.J. (2003) *A modern history of educating students with mild intellectual disabilities in Saskatchewan (1900–2002)*. M Ed. thesis. Saskatchewan: University of Saskatchewan.

Lakin, K.C. and Prouty, R. (2003) *Medicaid Home and Community-Based Services: The First 20 Years Policy*. Research Brief 14(3). University of Minnesota: Minneapolis, Institute on Community Integration.

Landes, D.S. (2003) *The Unbound Prometheus: Technological Change and Industrial Development in Western Europe from 1750 to the Present*, 2nd edn. Cambridge: Cambridge University Press.

Lanisef, P. and Lanphier, M. (2003) *The World in a City*. Toronto: University of Toronto Press.

Larson, S.A., Hewitt, A.S. and Lakin, K.C. (2004) Multiperspective analysis of workforce challenges and their effects on consumer and family quality of life. *American Journal on Mental Retardation*, 109(6): 481–500.

Lawhead, B. and Lawhead, A. (2007) Foreword, in D. Dileo. *Raymond's Room*. St Augustine, FL: Training Resource Network Inc.

Lawrence, K. and Crowther, C.A. (2003) Survey of current pre-natal screening for Down syndrome in Australian hospitals providing maternity care, *Australian and New Zealand Journal of Obstetrics and Gynaecology*, 43(3): 222–5.

Le Grand, J. and Bartlett, W. (eds) (1993) *Quasi-markets and Social Policy*. Basingstoke: Macmillan.

Lemay, R. (2006) Social role valorization insights into the social integration conundrum, *Mental Retardation*, 44(1): 1–12.

Lifton, R.J. (1986) *The Nazi Doctors: Medically Killing and Psychology of Genocide*. New York: Basic Books.

Lind, M. (1985) *Immigration, Migration and Settlement in the United States: A Genealogical Guidebook*. Minnesota: Linden Tree.

L'Institut Roeher Institute (1999) *Towards Inclusion: National Evaluation of Deinstitutionalization Initiatives*. Toronto: L'Institut Roeher Institute.

Lutfiyya, Z. (2005) *The three stages of inclusion*. Public lecture, University of Manitoba, 21 September.

Lyon, D. (2000) *Jesus in Disneyland: Religion in Postmodern Times*. Cambridge: Polity Press.

MacArthur, J. (2003) *Support of Daily Living for Adults with an Intellectual Disability: Review of the Literature Prepared for the National Advisory Committee on Health and Disability to Inform its Project on Services for Adults with an Intellectual Disability.* Wellington: NHC and Donald Beasley Institute.

McLaren, A. (1990) *Our Own Master Race: Eugenics in Canada, 1885–1945.* Toronto, Ontario: McClelland and Stewart.

McKnight, J. (1996) *The Careless Society: The Community and its Counterfeits.* Reprint Edition, New York: Basic Books.

Malin, N., Race, D. and Jones, G. (1980) *Services for the Mentally Handicapped in Britain.* London: Croom Helm.

Malin, N.A., Race, D.G., Manthorpe, J. and Wilmot, S. (1999) *Community Care for Nurses and the Caring Professions.* Buckingham: Open University Press.

Mansell, J., Beadle-Brown, J. and Clegg, S. (2004) The situation of large residential institutions in Europe, in G. Freyhoff, C. Parker, M. Coué and N. Greig (eds) *Included in Society: Results and Recommendations of the European Research Initiative on Community-based Residential Alternatives for Disabled People.* Brussels: Inclusion Europe, pp. 28–56.

May, D. (ed.) (2000) *Transition and Change in the Lives of People with Intellectual Disabilities.* London: Jessica Kingsley Publishers.

Meijer, C.J.W., Pijl, S.J. and Hegarty, S. (1997) Introduction, in S.J. Pijl, C.J.W. Meijer and S. Hegarty (eds) *Inclusive Education: A Global Agenda.* London: Routledge.

Mein Smith, P. (2005) *A Concise History of New Zealand.* Cambridge: Cambridge University Press.

Melnick, C. (2005) We can't close it yet, *Winnipeg Free Press*, 29 October

Menolascino, R., Clark, R.L. and Wolfensberger, W. (1968) *The Initiation and Development of a Comprehensive, County-wide System of Services for the Mentally Retarded of Douglas County*, 2nd edn. Vol. 1. Omaha, NE: Greater Omaha Association for Retarded Children.

Meyer, P. (2004) Goals, outcomes, and future challenges for people with intellectual disabilities in a noninstitutional society: the Norwegian experience, *Journal of Policy and Practice in Intellectual Disabilities*, 1(2): 95–102.

Mica (2005) *The Right to an Independent Life.* Ostersund, Mica.

Millen, J. (1999) *IHC's First 50 Years.* Wellington: IHC NZ Inc.

Millier, P. (1999) Normalization and Social Role Valorization in Australia and New Zealand, in R.J. Flynn and R.A. Lemay (eds) *A Quarter Century of Normalization and Social Role Valorization: Evolution and Impact.* Ottawa: University of Ottawa.

Minister for Disability Issues (2001) *New Zealand Disability Strategy.* Wellington: Office for Disability Issues.

Ministry of Community and Social Services (1987) *Challenges and Opportunities: Community Living for people with Developmental Handicaps.* Toronto.

Ministry of Education, Research and Church Affairs (1995) *On Education for children and adults with special needs.*

Mirfin-Veitch, B. (2003) *Education for Adults with an Intellectual Disability (Including Transition to Adulthood)*. Wellington: NHC and Donald Beasley Institute.

Mirfin-Veitch, B., Bray, A. and Ross, N. (2003) 'It was the hardest and most painful decision of my life!': seeking permanent out-of-home placement for sons and daughters with intellectual disabilities, *Journal of Intellectual & Developmental Disability*, 28(2): 9–111.

Miringoff, M. and Miringoff, M-L. (1999) *The Social Health of the Nation: How America Is Really Doing*. New York: Oxford University Press.

Mitchell, D.R. and Mitchell, J.W. (1985) *Out of the Shadows: A Chronology of Significant Events in the Development of Services for Exceptional Children and Young Persons in New Zealand, 1850–1983*. Wellington: Department of Education.

Mjoen J. A. (1914) *Rasehygiene*, 1st edn. Oslo: Jacob Dybwad.

Moen, T. (2003) Uten regler ville det blitt kaotisk. En studie av hvordan en lærer håndterer klasseromskompleksiteten. ['Without rules chaos rules': a study of how a teacher handles the complexity of the classroom], in M.B. Postholm, and T. Pettersson (eds) *Klasseledelse [Classroom Management]*. Oslo: Universitetsforlaget, pp. 111–28.

Moen, T. (2004) *Kids need to be seen: a narrative study of a teacher's inclusive education*. Unpublished Dr Polit Thesis, Department of Education, Norwegian University of Science and Technology, NTNU, Trondheim.

Moen, T. and Gudmundsdottir, S. (1997) *Det å send han Tom ut av klassen, e ikkje nån løysning. En kasusstudie av inkluderende prosesser. ['Kicking Tom out of the classroom is no solution'. A Case Study of Inclusive Processes]*. Trondheim: Tapir.

Moore, A. and Tennant, M. (1997) *Who Is Responsible for the Provision of Support Services for People with Disabilities?* Wellington: National Health Committee, pp. 1–50.

Mordal, K.N. and Strømstad, M. (1998) Adapted education for some? in T. Booth and M. Ainscow (eds) *From Them to Us: International Study of Inclusion in Education*. London & New York: Routledge.

Morris, J. (1991) *Pride Against Prejudice: Transforming Attitudes to Disability*. London: The Women's Press.

Morris, J. (2005) *Independent living: the role of evidence and ideology in the development of government policy*. Paper delivered at Cash and Care Conference, Social Policy Research Unit, University of York, 12–13 April.

Morris, P. (1969) *Put Away: A Sociological Study of Institutions for the Mentally Retarded*. London: Routledge and Kegan Paul.

Moseley, C., Gettings, R. and Cooper, R. (2003) *Having It Your Way: Understanding State Individual Budgeting Strategies Survey for National Association of State Directors of Developmental Disabilities Services (NASDDDS)*. Alexandria, VA: NASDDDS.

Munford, R. and Sullivan, M. (1997) Social theories of disability: the insurrection of subjugated knowledges, in P. O'Brien and R. Murray (eds) *Human*

Services: Towards Partnership and Support. Palmerston North: The Dunmore Press Ltd.

Murray, M. (1994) *Losing Ground: American Social Policy 1950–1980,* 10th anniversary edition. New York: Basic Books.

National Center for Special Education Research (NCSER) (2006) *An Overview of Findings from Wave 2 of the National Longitudinal Transition Study–2 (NLTS2).* NCSER, Institute of Educational Sciences.

National Geographic (2007) *The Genographic Project.* https://www3.nationalgeographic.com/genographic/atlas.html?fs=www3.nationalgeographic.com (accessed 08/01/07).

National Health Committee (NHC) (2003) *To Have an 'Ordinary' Life: Kia whai oranga 'noa'.* Wellington: NHC.

National Institute for Clinical Excellence (NICE) (2003) *Antenatal Care: Routine Care for the Healthy Woman.* London: NICE.

National Institute on Mental Retardation. (NIMR) (1974) *A Plan for Comprehensive Community Services for the Developmentally Handicapped (ComServ).* Toronto: Canadian Association for the Mentally Retarded.

New York State (NYS) (undated) *Your Family Rights: A Family Guide for the New York State Early Intervention Program for Infants and Toddlers with Disabilities.* Albany, NY: NYS Department of Health and NYS Commission on Quality of Care for the Mentally Disabled.

New York State Education Department (2002) *Special Education in New York State for Children Ages 3–21: A Parent's Guide.* Albany, NY: New York State Education Department and The University of the State of New York.

New Zealand Institute on Mental Retardation (1980) *Standards for Residential Services.* Wellington: NZMR.

Nirje, B. (1969) The Normalization principle and its human management implications, in R. B. Kugel and W. Wolfensberger (eds) *Changing Patterns in Residential Services for the Mentally Retarded.* Washington, DC: President's Committee on Mental Retardation, US Government Printing Office.

Nirje, B. (1999) How I came to formulate the Normalization Principle, in R.J. Flynn and R.A. Lemay (eds) *A Quarter Century of Normalization and Social Role Valorization: evolution and impact.* Ottawa: University of Ottawa.

Noll, S. and Trent, J.W. Jnr. (eds) (2004) *Mental Retardation in America: A Historical Reader.* New York: New York University Press.

North Carolina Council On Developmental Disabilities (NCCDD) (2007) Flyer for *'Service Transformation: When Person-Centered Options are Made Available to All People Served. . . . Without Exception.* www.nccdd.org

NOU (Official Norwegian Report) 1985:34 (1985) *Levekår for psykisk utviklingshemmede [Living conditions for mentally retarded].* Oslo: Det Kongelige Sosialdepartement.

O'Brien, C.L., O'Brien, J. and Mount, B. (1997) Person-centered planning has arrived . . . Or has it? *Mental Retardation,* 480–4.

O'Brien, C.L. and O'Brien, J. (2000) *The Origins of Person-Centred Planning: A Community of Practice Perspective*. Georgia: Responsive Systems Associates.

O'Brien, J. (2005a) *Reflecting on Social Roles: Identifying Opportunities to Support Personal Freedom and Social Integration Through Wisconsin's Restructuring Initiative*. Georgia: Responsive Systems Associates.

O'Brien, J. (2005b) *'. . . to Interact with Non-disabled Persons to the Fullest Extent Possible'. Perspectives On 'Most Integrated' Services for People with Developmental Disabilities*. Georgia: Responsive Systems Associates.

O'Brien, J., Carssow, K., Jones, M., Mercer, M., Reynolds, L. and Strzok, D. (2003) *Never Give Up: Asset Inc.'s Commitment to Community Life for People seen as 'Difficult to Serve'*. Anchorage: Assets, Inc.

O'Brien, J. and Forest, M. (1989) *Action for Inclusion*. Toronto: Inclusion Press.

O'Brien, J. and O'Brien, C. L. (2006) *'And Now They Need A Life': A Formative Evaluation of Wisconsin's Money Follows the Person Grant as it Influenced Services for People with Developmental Disabilities*. Wisconsin.

O'Brien, J., O'Brien, C.L. and Jacob, G. (1998) *Celebrating the Ordinary*. Toronto: Inclusion Press.

O'Brien, P. (2005). Returning to one's roots: Haki Titori's story, in K. Johnson and R. Traustadottir (eds) *Deinstitutionalization and People with Intellectual Disabilities*. London: Jessica Kingsley Publishers.

O'Brien, P. and Murray, R. (eds) (1997) *Human Services: Towards Partnership and Support*. Palmerston North, NZ: The Dunmore Press Ltd.

O'Brien, P. and Ryba, K. (2005) Policies and practices in special education, in D. Fraser, R. Moltzen and K. Ryba (eds) *Learners with Special Needs in Aotearoa/New Zealand*, 3rd edn. Southbank, Victoria: Thomson Dunmore Press.

Odin (2007) http://odin.dep.no/hod/english/bn.html

Office for Disability Issues (ODI) (2005) *Briefing to the Incoming Minister: Making a World of Difference*. Wellington: ODI.

Office for Disability Issues (ODI) (2006) *UN Convention on Rights of Disabled People*. http://www.odi.govt.nz/what-we-do/un-convention.html (accessed 26/01/07).

Office of Disability (1991, 1997, 2003) *Agreement between THE COMMONWEALTH OF AUSTRALIA and THE STATES AND TERRITORIES OF AUSTRALIA in Relation to Disability Services*. Canberra: Office of Disability.

Olmstead v L.C (1999) http://www.bazelon.org/issues/disabilityrights/incourt/olmstead/index.htm (accessed 30/01/07).

O'Shane (1995) Opening address to Australian Society for the Study of Intellectual Disability (ASSID) Conference, Melbourne, October, reprinted in O'Brien and Murray (1997).

Oshel.com (2007) *History of International Migration*. http://www.oshel.com/history_of_international_migrati.htm (accessed 26/01/07).

PASC (2007) *Work Opportunities for 15–19 Year-Olds*, Leaflet from PASC, Calgary, Alberta.

Patton, J.M. (1998) The disproportionate representation of African Americans in special education: looking behind the curtain for understanding and solutions, *The Journal of Special Education*, 32: 25–31.

Pearpoint, J., O'Brien, J. and Forest, M. (1993) *Path: Planning Possible Positive Futures*, 2nd edn. Toronto: Inclusion Press.

Pelly, M. (2005) Life, death and responsibility under the gavel *Sydney Morning Herald*, 11/11/05.

People First http://www.peoplefirst.org.uk/pflinks.html

Peterson, N. and Sanders, W. (eds) (1998) *Citizenship and Indigenous Australians: Changing Conceptions and Possibilities*. Cambridge and Melbourne: Cambridge University Press.

Pettersson, T. (2000) *Det levende ordet i en krevende klasse [The Living Word in a Demanding Classroom]*. Trondheim: Tapir.

Pilcher, J. and Wagg, S. (1996) *Thatcher's Children?: Politics, Childhood and Society in the 1980s and 1990s*. Abingdon: RoutledgeFalmer.

Posner, S.F., Learman, L.A., E.A. Gates, E.A., Washington, A.E. and Kuppermann, M. (2004) Development of an attitudes measure for pre-natal screening in diverse populations, *Social Indicators Research*, 65(2): 187–206(20).

Powell, M. (ed.) (2002) *Evaluating New Labour's Welfare Reforms*. Bristol: Policy Press.

Progressive Alternatives Society of Calgary *Youth Employment Source (YES)*. http://www.pasc-calgary.org/ (accessed 27/01/07).

Prouty, R.W., Smith, G. and Lakin, C. (eds) (2006) *Residential Services for Persons with Developmental Disabilities: Status and Trends Through 2005*. Minneapolis: Research and Training Centeron Community Living, University of Minnesota.

Putnam, R. (2000) *Bowling Alone: The Collapse and Revival of American Community*. New York: Simon and Schuster.

Queensland Parents for People with a Disability (QPPD) (2001) *Education Queensland's Placement Policy and Process*. Paddington, Queensland: QPPD.

Queensland Parents for People with a Disability (QPPD) (2003) *There's Small Choice in Rotten Apples: An Exploration of the Process of Parental Decision-making around Educational Choice for Parents of Children with Disabilities*. Paddington, Queensland: QPPD.

Queensland Parents for People with a Disability (QPPD) (2005) *The Pendulum is Swinging Back: An Evaluation of the Challenges in the Lives of People with Disabilities*. Paddington, Queensland: QPPD.

Race, D.G. (1977) *Investigation into the effects of different caring environments on the social competence of mentally handicapped adults*. Unpublished PhD thesis: University of Reading.

Race, D.G. (1999) *Social Role Valorization and the English Experience*. London: Wilding and Birch.

Race, D.G. (2002a) *Learning Disability: A Social Approach*. London: Routledge.

Race, D.G. (2002b) 'The Historical Context', in D. G. Race (ed.) *Learning Disability: A Social Approach*. London: Routledge.

Race, D.G. (2002c) The 'Normalisation' debate – time to move on, in D. G. Race (ed.) *Learning Disability: A Social Approach*. London: Routledge.

Race, D.G. (2003) *Leadership and Change in Human Services: Selected Readings from Wolf Wolfensberger*. London: Routledge.

Race, D.G. (2005) Learning disability, housing and community care, in M. Foord and P. Simic (eds) *Housing, Community Care and Supported Housing – Resolving Contradictions*. Coventry: Chartered Institute of Housing, Coventry.

Race, D.G. (2007) A tale of two White Papers, *Journal of Intellectual Disabilities*, 11(1): 83–103.

Race, D.G., Boxall, K. and Carson, I. (2005) Same difference? The impact of Social Role Valorization and the social model of disability on service delivery and individualised support for people with learning difficulties, *Disability and Society*, 20(5): 507–21.

Race, D.G. and Race, D.M. (1978) Services for the mentally handicapped in Sweden, *Child: Care, Health and Development*, 4(3): 183–94.

Race, D.G. and Race, D.M. (1979) *The Cherries Group Home: A Beginning*. London: HMSO.

Race, D.G. and Williams, P. (1988) *Normalisation and the Children's Society*. London: CMHERA.

Race, D.M. (2006) Partnership working in learning disability services: an exploration, unpublished MSc thesis submitted to Health Services Management Centre, University of Birmingham.

Ramcharan, P., Roberts, G., Grant, G. and Borland, J. (1997) *Empowerment in Everyday Life: Learning Disability*. London: Jessica Kingsley.

Ramsey, S. (2005) *Roles Based Planning: A Thoughtful Approach to Social Inclusion AND Empowerment*. Calgary: DDRC & everyone belongs.

Raper, M. (2000) *Public and private sector roles in social services*. Paper to 29th ICSW international conference: Cape Town, 23–27 October. http://www.icsw.org/global-conferences/public-private-sector-role.htm (accessed 25/01/07).

Rees, S. and G. Rodley (eds) (1995) *The Human Cost of Managerialism*. Sydney: Pluto.

Rescare New Zealand (2007) http://www.rescarenz.com/ (accessed 26/01/07).

Reschly, D.J. (1997) *Disproportionate Minority Representation in General and Special Education: Patterns, Issues and Alternatives*. Des Moines, IA: Mountain Plains Regional Resource Center, Drake University.

Retsinas, K. (1991) Impact of pre-natal technology on attitudes toward disabled infants, in D. Wertz (ed.) *Research in the Sociology of Healthcare*. Westport, CT: JAI Press, pp. 75–102.

Ringsby-Jansson, B. (2002) *Arenas of Everyday Life: About People with Intellectual Disabilities and their Everyday and Social Life*. Goteborg: Institutionen for social arbete, Goteborgs universiteit.

Rizzolo, M.C., Hemp, R., Braddock, D. and Pomeranz-Essley, A. (2004) *The State of the States*. Washington, DC: American Association on Mental Retardation (AAMR).

Roll-Hansen, N. (1996) Norwegian eugenics: sterilization as social reform, in G. Broberg and N. Roll-Hansen (eds) *Eugenics and the Welfare State: Sterilization Policy in Denmark, Sweden, Norway and Finland*. East Lansing, MI: Michigan State University Press.

Rollo, J. (2005) Post-school programs for adults with intellectual disability: an Australian example, A presentation at the International Cornelia de Lange Syndrome Conference, Grosseto, Italy, 18 June 2005.

Romøren, T. I. (1995) *HVPU-reformen i forskningens lys [HVPUreform in the light of research]*. Oslo: Ad Notam Gyldendal.

Rosenau, N. (2000) Do we really mean families for all children? Permanency planning for children with developmental disabilities. Policy Research Brief 11 (2), 1–12, University of Minnesota, Minneapolis, Institute on Community Integration.

Rothman, S. and Rothman, D. (2005) *The Willowbrook Wars*. New Brunswick, NJ: Aldine Transaction.

Runcis, M. (1998) *Sterilisation in the Swedish Welfare State*. Stockholm University. Ardfront: Stockholm.

Rustemier, S. and Vaughan, M. (2005) *Are LEAs in England Abandoning Inclusive Education?* London: CSIE.

Ryan, J. and Thomas, F. (1987) *The Politics of Mental Handicap*, 2nd edn. Harmondsworth: Penguin.

S&S Consultants (2005) *Achieving the vision: transitions and participation – considering the opportunities*. A discussion paper prepared for the Australian Government May 2005.

Sabe USA http://www.sabeusa.org/

Saetersdal B. (1994) *Menneskeskjebner i HPVU-reformenstid (Human Fortunes in the Era of Deinstituionalization)*. Oslo: Universitetsforlaget.

Sanderson, H., Duffy, S., Poll, C. and Hatton, C. (2006) In Control: the story so far, *Journal of Integrated Care* 14(4): 3–13.

Saunders, P. (2005) *The impact of disability on living standards: reviewing Australian evidence and policies*. Presentation to the Cash and Care: Understanding the Evidence Base for Policy and Practice Conference, SPRU, University of York 12, 13 April.

Savage, M. (2000) *Class Analysis and Social Transformation*. Milton Keynes: Open University Press.

Schalock, R.L. (ed.) (2002) *Out of the Darkness, into the Light: Nebraska's Experience with Mental Retardation*. Washington, DC: AAMR.

Scheerenberger, R.C. (1987) *A History of Mental Retardation*. Baltimore, MD: Brookes.

SDV (*Samhallsintegrerad Daglig Verksamhet*) (2005) *Informationsfolder*. Jonkoping: Jonkopings Kommun.

Seierstad, S. (1998) Utsyn over statlige og kommunale attforingstiltak (Review of labour market programmes for people with occupational disabilities), in

S. Seierstad, A.K. Eide, K.M. Helle and A. Schaft (eds) *Evaluering av de statlige arbeidssamvirketiltakene og de kommunale aktivitetstilbudene for yrkeshemmede (Evaluating state and municipal labour market programmes)*. Oslo: AFIs rapportserie 5/98.

Senate Committee (2002) *Education of Students with Disabilities*. Canberra: Senate Employment, Workplace Relations and Education References Committee.

Shakespeare, T. (2006) *Disability Rights and Wrongs*. London: Routledge.

Shaw, L. (1990) *Each Belongs: Integrated Education in Canada*. Bristol: Centre for Studies on Inclusive Education (CSIE).

Sherwin, J. (2005) Hope, in L. Shevallar, S. Pacey and P Collins (eds) *On Being the Change We Want to See*. Brisbane: CRU.

Shevallar, L., Pacey, S. and Collins, P. (eds) (2005) *On Being the Change We Want To See*. Brisbane: CRU.

Simon, B. (1991) *Education and the Social Order: British Education Since 1944*. Basingstoke: Palgrave Macmillan.

Singer, G. and Powers, L. (1993) *Families, Disability and Empowerment*. Baltimore MD: Brookes.

Socialstyrelsen (2006) *Measures under the Act Concerning Support and Service for Persons with Certain Functional Impairments (LSS)*. Stockholm: National Board of Health and Welfare, Socialstyrelsen Art. no 2006–114–16.

Statistics Canada (2001) *Participation and Activity Limitations Survey*. Ottawa: Statistics Canada.

Stone, P. and Austin, D. (2004) *Assessment of Antenatal Screening for Down Syndrome in New Zealand*. Auckland: Auckland UniServices Ltd.

Special Education (2000) *Monitoring and Evaluation of the Policy – Phase 3, Final Report*. Wellington, NZ: Ministry of Education.

SOU (Swedish Government Official Reports) 1946:24 *Forslag till effektiviserad kurators – och arbetsformedlingsverksamhet for partiellt arbetsfora m m*. Stockholm.

St. Meld (1967) *Ansvar for tiltak og tenester for psykiske utviklingshemma*, 67: 86–87. Oslo: Sosialdepartementet.

Sullivan, L. (2001) *Paper to Auckland Provider Network Forum 22/06/01*. Auckland: access ability.

Taylor. S. J. (2005) The institutions are dying, but are not dead yet, in K. Johnson, and R. Traustadottir (eds) *Deinstitutionalization and People with Intellectual Disabilities*. London: Jessica Kingsley Publishers.

Thatcher, M. (1987) talking to *Women's Own* magazine, October 31 1987, as quoted on http://briandeer.com/social/thatcher-society.htm (accessed 18/11/05).

Thompson, E.P. (1991) *The Making of the English Working Class*. London: Penguin Books.

Tideman, M. (2005) Conquering life: the experiences of the first integrated generation, in K. Johnson and R Traustadottir (eds) *Deinstitutionalization and People with Intellectual Disabilities*. London: Jessica Kingsley Publishers.

Tideman, M. and Tøssebro, J. (2002) A comparison of living conditions for intellectually disabled people in Norway and Sweden: following the national reforms in the 1990s, *Scandinavian Journal of Disability Research*, 4: 23–42.

Tøssebro, J. (1992) *Institusjonsliv i velferdsstaten (Institutions in the Welfare State)*. Oslo: ad Notam Gyldendal.

Tøssebro, J. (1996) *En bedre hverdag? Utviklingshemmetes levekar etter HVPU-reformen (A better life? Intellectually Disabled People's Living Conditions after Relocation from Institutions)*. Oslo: Kommuneforlaget.

Tøssebro, J. (2005) Reflections on living outside: continuity and change in the life of 'outsiders', in K. Johnson, and R. Traustadottir (ed.) *Deinstitutionalization and People with Intellectual Disabilities*. London: Jessica Kingsley Publishers.

Tøssebro, J. and Lundeby, H. (2002) *Statlig reform og communal hverdag: Utviklingshemmetes levekar ti ar etter reformen (State Reform and Local Practice: Living Conditions of Intellectually Disabled People Ten Years after Resettlement)*. Trondheim: Norwegian University of Science and Technology.

Traustadottir, R. (2006) *Disability studies: a Nordic perspective*. A seminar presented on 17 May at the Centre for Applied Disability Studies, University of Sheffield.

Tredgold, A.F. (1909) The feebleminded – a social danger, *Eugenics Review*, 1: 97–104.

Tredgold, A.F. (1952) *A Textbook on Mental Deficiency (Amentia)*, 8th edn. London: Bailliere, Tindall & Cox.

Trent J.W. Jnr. (1994) *Inventing the Feebleminded: A History of Mental Retardation in the United States* Berkeley: University of California Press.

Trevelyan, G.M. (2000) *English Social History*. London: Penguin Books.

Tse, E. (1984) The myth of sheltered employment, *Australian Disability Review*, 1: 16–21.

United Nations (2006) *Human Development Index (HDI)* http://hdr.undp.org/hdr2006/statistics/indicators/10.html (accessed 23/01/07).

U.S. Department of Education (2003) *To Assure the Free Appropriate Public Education of All Children With Disabilities: The Twenty-fifth Annual Report to Congress on the Implementation of the Individuals With Disabilities Education Act*. Washington, DC: U.S. Government Printing Office.

Valuing People Support Team (2005) *The Government's Annual Report on Learning Disability 2005 – Valuing People: Making Things Better*. Cmnd 6700. London: The Stationery Office.

Valuing People Website (Tools for modernising day services) http://valuingpeople.gov.uk/dynamic/valuingpeople117.jsp

Van Kraayenoord, C., Elkins, J., Palmer, C., Rickards, F.W. and Colbert, E. (2000) *Literacy, Numeracy and Students with Disabilities*. Canberra ACT: Department of Education, Training and Youth Affairs (DETYA).

Vogt, R. (1914) *Avrelighetslaere og Racehygiene Kristiania*. Oslo: Cammermeyer.

Waerness, K. (2005) *Research on care: what impact on policy and planning?* Paper delivered at Cash and Care Conference, Social Policy Research Unit, University of York, 12–13 April.

Weber, M. (2005) *The Protestant Ethic and the Spirit of Capitalism: and Other Writings*. London: Longman.

Westcott, R. (2003) *Lives Unrealised: Clienthood and the Disability Industry*. Canberra: The Australian Institute on Intellectual Disability.

Wikipedia (2006) *Abortion in Canada*. http://en.wikipedia.org/wiki/Abortion-_in_Canada (accessed 16/11/06).

Wikipedia (2007) *Snoezelen*. http://en.wikipedia.org/wiki/Snoezelen (accessed 25/01/07).

Wills, D. (2005) Trends in Australian education: the inclusion of children with labels, in *The Challenge of Inclusion: People labeled with 'Challenging Behaviour' and the Struggle to Belong – Conference Papers 2005*. Brisbane: Community Resource Unit.

Wolfensberger, W. (1970) Models of mental retardation, *New Society*, 15(380): 51–3.

Wolfensberger, W. (1972) *Normalization: The Principle of Normalization in Human Services*, Toronto: National Institute on Mental Retardation.

Wolfensberger, W. (1983) Social Role Valorization: a proposed new term for the principle of normalization, *Mental Retardation*, 21(6): 234–9.

Wolfensberger, W. (1984) A reconceptualization of normalization as social role valorization, *Mental Retardation (Canada)*, 34(7): 22–6.

Wolfensberger, W. (1998) *A Brief Introduction to Social Role Valorisation: A High-order Concept for Addressing the Plight of Societally Devalued People, and for Structuring Human Services*, 3rd edn., (Rev.) Syracuse, NY: Syracuse University, Training Institute for Human Service Planning, Leadership and Change Agency.

Wolfensberger, W. (1999) A contribution to the history of normalization, with primary emphasis on the establishment of normalization in North America between 1967–1975, in R.J. Flynn and R.A. Lemay (eds) *A Quarter Century of Normalization and Social Role Valorization: Evolution and Impact*. Ottawa: University of Ottawa Press.

Wolfensberger, W. (2002) Social Role Valorization and, or versus 'empowerment', *Mental Retardation*, 40: 252–8.

Wolfensberger, W. and Glenn, L. (1975, reprinted 1978) *Program Analysis of Service Systems (PASS): A Method for the Quantitative Evaluation of Human Services*, Vol. 2. Field manual, 3rd edn. Toronto: National Institute on Mental Retardation.

Wolfensberger, W. and Thomas, S. (1983) *PASSING (Program Analysis of Service Systems' Implementation of Normalization Goals): Normalization Criteria and ratings Manual*, 2nd edn. Toronto: National Institute on Mental Retardation.

Wolfensberger, W., Thomas, S. and Caruso, G. (1996) Some of the universal 'good things of life' which the implementation of Social Role Valorization can be expected to make more accessible to devalued people, *SRV/VRS: The International Social Role Valorization Journal/La Revue Internationale de la Valorisation des Roles Sociaux* 2(2): 12–14.

Legislation

Australia

Disability Discrimination Act 1992
States Grant (Primary and Secondary Education Assistance) Act 2000

Canada

The Constitution Act 1867 previously known as the British North America Act of 1867
Developmental Services Act 1974.

England

Mental Deficiency Act 1913
Education Act 1944
National Health Services Act 1946
Mental Health Act 1959
Education (Handicapped Children) Act 1970
Education Act 1981
Community Care (Direct Payments) Act 1986
NHS and Community Care Act 1990
Abortion (Amendment) Act 1990
Disability Discrimination Act 1995
The Community Care (Direct Payments) Act 1996
Local Government Act 1999
Health Services Act 2000
Education Act 2002
Education Act 2005

New Zealand

The Mental Defectives Act 1911
Mental Health Act 1954
Mental Health Act 1956
Crimes Act 1961 (with amendments in 1977 and 1978)
The Contraception, Sterilisation, and Abortion Act 1977 (CS&A)
State Sector Act 1988
Injury Prevention, Rehabilitation and Compensation Act 2001
Care of Children Act 2004

Norway

The Education of Abnormal Children Act 1881
The Abortion Law 1975
Act relating to Primary and Secondary Education (Education Act). Last amended 17 June 2005.

Sweden

Act for Services to the Mentally Retarded 1967
Act on Special Services for Developmentally Disabled Persons 1986
Assistance Benefit Act (LASS) 1993
Special Act on Supports and Services for Persons With Certain Functional Impairments (LSS) 1994
Abolition of Institutions Act 1997
Social Services Act 2002

United States of America

Education for all Handicapped Children Act of 1975
No Child Left Behind Act 2001
Individuals with Disabilities Education Improvement Act of 2004

Index

Related books from Open University Press

Purchase from www.openup.co.uk or order through your local bookseller

---

LEARNING DISABILITY
A LIFE CYCLE APPROACH TO VALUING PEOPLE

Gordon Grant, Peter Goward, Malcolm Richardson
and Paul Ramcharan

This practical and accessible key text examines the nature and impact of collaboration between different professional and voluntary groups working together to deliver
services. The first section explores partnership in terms of language, politics, diversity,
user perspectives, rurality and ethics. In section two, carefully selected authors draw
upon their expertise to raise key questions, and use case studies to demonstrate the
challenges of working in partnership in areas where collaboration is a crucial to effective practice, this includes: child protection; drug using parents; dementia; travelling
families; domestic violence; learning difficulties; homelessness; mentally disordered
offenders; HIV and AIDS; disaffected youth, and older people.

This book is recommended reading for managers, practitioners and students from a
variety of human service agencies – it will provide good understanding into issues,
pitfalls and best practice to work effectively in partnership with other agencies. A must
read for anyone about to develop or join a multi agency partnership.

Contributors
Althea Allison; John Bates; Liz Blyth; Julian Buchanan; Ros Carnwell; Alex Carson; Pat
Chambers; Michael Clark; Brian Corby; Jacquie Evans; Ian Iles; David Jolley; Thoby
Miller; Amir Minhas; Virginia Minogue; Neil Moreland; Lester Parrott; Judith Phillips;
Richard Pugh; Kate Read; Angela Roberts; Debbie Williams; Ruth Wilson; Ruth Wyner

Contents
*Acknowledgements – About the Editors – List of Contributors – Preface – Part One:
The Construction of Learning Disability – Part Two: Childhood: Rights, Risks & Responsi-
bilities – Part Three: Independence: Adolescents and the Younger Adult – Part Four: Social
Inclusion and Adulthood – Part Five: Citizenship and the Older Adult – Index*

2005   784pp
ISBN-13: 978 0 335 21439 6 (ISBN-10: 0 335 21439 8) Paperback
ISBN-13: 978 0 335 21864 4 (ISBN-10: 0 335 21826 1) Hardback

EFFECTIVE PRACTICE IN HEALTH AND SOCIAL CARE
Ros Carnwell and Julian Buchanan

This practical and accessible key text examines the nature and impact of collaboration between different professional and voluntary groups working together to deliver services. The first section explores partnership in terms of language, politics, diversity, user perspectives, rurality and ethics. In section two, carefully selected authors draw upon their expertise to raise key questions, and use case studies to demonstrate the challenges of working in partnership in areas where collaboration is a crucial to effective practice, this includes: child protection; drug using parents; dementia; travelling families; domestic violence; learning difficulties; homelessness; mentally disordered offenders; HIV and AIDS; disaffected youth, and older people.

This book is recommended reading for managers, practitioners and students from a variety of human service agencies – it will provide good understanding into issues, pitfalls and best practice to work effectively in partnership with other agencies. A must read for anyone about to develop or join a multi agency partnership.

Contributors
Althea Allison; John Bates; Liz Blyth; Julian Buchanan; Ros Carnwell; Alex Carson; Pat Chambers; Michael Clark; Brian Corby; Jacquie Evans; Ian Iles; David Jolley; Thoby Miller; Amir Minhas; Virginia Minogue; Neil Moreland; Lester Parrott; Judith Phillips; Richard Pugh; Kate Read; Angela Roberts; Debbie Williams; Ruth Wilson; Ruth Wyner

Contents

2004   304pp
ISBN-13: 978 0 335 21437 2 (ISBN-10: 0 335 21437 1) Paperback
ISBN-13: 978 0 335 21438 9 (ISBN-10: 0 335 21438 X) Hardback

WORKING WITH CHILDREN IN CARE
EUROPEAN PERSPECTIVES

Pat Petrie, Janet Boddy, Valerie Wigfall and Claire Cameron

- How does residential care in England compare with that of other European countries?
- What is social pedagogy, and how does it help those working with children in care?
- How can child care policy and practice be improved throughout the United Kingdom?

This book is written against the background of the gross social disadvantage suffered by most looked-after children in England. It compares European policy and approaches – from Belgium, Denmark, France, Germany and the Netherlands – to the public care system in England. Drawing on research from all six countries, the authors analyze how different policies and practice can affect young people in residential homes. A particular focus is on the unique approach offered by social pedagogy, a concept that is commonly used in continental Europe.

The book compares young people's own experiences and appraisals of living in a residential home, and the extent to which residential care compounds social exclusion. Based upon theoretical and empirical evidence, it offers solutions for current dilemmas concerning looked-after children in the United Kingdom, in terms of lessons learned from policy and practice elsewhere, including training and staffing issues.

Working with Children in Care is key reading for students, academics and professionals in health, education and social care who work with children in residential care.

Contents
Introduction – What is pedagogy? – National differences in policy and training for work with looked after children – Working in residential care – Understandings and values: Staff responses to hypothetical situations – Looked-after lives – Giving children a good start? – Policy and practice in England: What is it in our current situation that makes it difficult to do well? – Concluding discussion, lessons learned – Appendix

2006   208pp
ISBN-13: 978 0 335 21634 5 (ISBN-10: 0 335 21634 X) Paperback
ISBN-13: 978 0 335 21635 2 (ISBN-10: 0 335 21635 8) Hardback

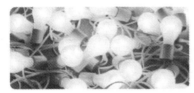 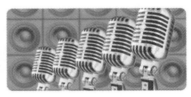
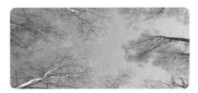 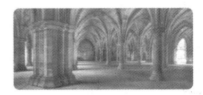
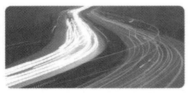 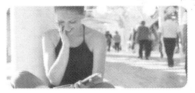
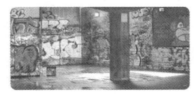
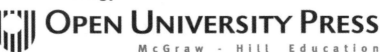
UNIVERSITY OF WOLVERHAMPTON
LEARNING & INFORMATION SERVICES